Successful Communication with Alzheimer's Disease Patients

Successful Communication with Alzheimer's Disease Patients

An In-Service Training Manual

Mary Jo Santo Pietro, Ph.D. CCC-s
*Associate Professor of Speech Pathology, and
Director, Speech and Hearing Clinic, Kean College
of New Jersey, Union*

Elizabeth Ostuni, M.A. CCC-s
Director, Accent on Communication, Sparta, NJ

Butterworth–Heinemann
Boston   Oxford   Johannesburg   Melbourne   New Delhi   Singapore

Butterworth–Heinemann supports the efforts of American Forests and the Global ReLeaf Program in its campaign for the betterment of trees, forests, and our environment.

Library of Congress Cataloging-in-Publication Data

Santo Pietro, Mary Jo Cook, 1945–
    Successful communication with Alzheimer's disease patients : an in
-service training manual / Mary Jo Santo Pietro, Elizabeth
Ostuni.
      p.   cm.
    Includes bibliographical references and index.
    ISBN 0-7506-9564-1
    1. Alzheimer's disease--Nursing--Psychological aspects.
2. Interpersonal communication. 3. Alzheimer's disease--Patients-
-Nursing home care. I. Ostuni, Elizabeth. II. Title.
    [DNLM: 1. Alzheimer's Disease--nurses' instruction.
2. Communication--nurses' instruction. 3. Inservice Training.   WT
155 S237s 1997]
RC523.S27   1997
616.8'31--dc21
DNLM/DLC
for Library of Congress   96-54719
                                                 CIP

British Library Cataloguing-in-Publication Data
A catalogue record for this book is available from the British Library.

The publisher offers special discounts on bulk orders of this book.
For information, please contact:

Manager of Special Sales
Butterworth–Heinemann
313 Washington Street
Newton, MA 02158–1626
Tel: 617-928-2500
Fax: 617-928-2620

For information on all medical publications available, contact our World Wide Web home page at: http://www.bh.com/med

10 9 8 7 6 5 4 3 2 1

Printed in the United States of America

To Lilly Miller, whose dedication to the ongoing training of nursing home professionals is without equal: Thank you for so kindly supporting us in the presentation of our workshops over the years.

A Living Will

When they say I cannot
hear you, sing me lullabies
and folk songs, the ones
I sang to you. I will hear them
as an unborn child can hear
its mother's music through
the waters of the womb.

When they say I can feel
nothing, press your face
against my forehead, rest your
hand against my cheek. I
will feel them as the woman
at the window feels the wind
outside the glass.

When they say I'm past
all caring, brush my hair
and braid in ribbons. I will
know it as the seashells
on my table know the
rhythms of the sea.

When they tell you
to go home, stay with me
if you can. Deep
inside I will be
weeping.

—Naomi Halperin Spigle

(Reprinted with permission from SH Martz [ed], I Am Becoming the Woman
I've Wanted. Watsonville, CA: Papier-Mache Press, 1995;216.)

Contents

Preface

Human beings use more than words to communicate. Tone of voice, gestures, the clothes we wear, and the way we decorate our homes also send messages about what we think and how we feel. Yet even with all these avenues of expression available, we often struggle to find the right words or to understand a coworker's meaning. The challenge is far greater when we are expected to communicate with Alzheimer's disease patients who have major communication disorders.

Nevertheless, better communication with both coworkers and patients is a worthwhile goal. It is also an achievable one. As speech-language pathologists, we have spent many years working directly with Alzheimer's disease patients, researching their communication disorders, and presenting our findings in workshops to colleagues, professional caregivers, and administrators. We began to realize that these same lectures and workshops could be redesigned as in-service units and used more economically in on-site training programs. We have compiled a comprehensive and practical handbook filled with hundreds of proven techniques. These techniques have been drawn from numerous research articles and texts, and from our own extensive clinical experience.

Successful Communication with Alzheimer's Disease Patients is a series of in-service units written especially for professionals who care for persons with Alzheimer's disease. Every unit focuses on a specific aspect of communication in long-term care settings. Each unit recommends effective techniques that show how to become a better communicator, how to support patients' best communication efforts, and how to minimize or avoid disastrous communication breakdowns.

In any nursing home, there are at least four groups who would find this manual especially helpful for improving job performance: (1) *instructors* who need materials and information for conducting in-service programs for Alzheimer's disease patient caregivers, (2) *in-service participants* who will use the text and activities to improve their skills in caring for persons with severe communication limitations, (3) *individual staff members or volunteers* who wish to learn more about caring for patients with dementia but who do not have in-service programs available, and (4) *supervisors and administrators* who wish to understand and institute a high standard of communication skill throughout the organization.

However, *Successful Communication with Alzheimer's Disease Patients* is not directed exclusively to nursing home personnel. This handbook is an excellent resource for employees and volunteers in any setting in which elderly patients and demented patients spend their time—private homes, group homes, adult day-care centers, and rehabilitation hospitals. Finally, we propose that this material be used by educators in direct care staff certification programs and in university departments of gerontology where caregiving practices and ethics are shaped.

GOALS OF *SUCCESSFUL COMMUNICATION WITH ALZHEIMER'S DISEASE PATIENTS*

The primary purpose of *Successful Communication with Alzheimer's Disease Patients* is to make the job of professional caregiver easier, more efficient, and more pleasant. Improving communication skills between caregiver and patient, as well as between coworkers, is an important step toward increasing overall job satisfaction. The communication principles and practices introduced in this manual should reinforce the feeling that professional caregiving is a positive career choice.

The second purpose of *Successful Communication with Alzheimer's Disease Patients* is to show how effective communication practices foster an institutional environment in which patients are happier and more compliant. Our observation has been that if all persons employed in a facility improve their communication skills, the quality of caregiving that each resident receives improves markedly. In other words, "Good communication is good caregiving."*

A third purpose is to provide a missing link of information and skills that most formal education programs neglect and most nursing home jobs require—the basic "how-to" of communicating with residents who have Alzheimer's disease. In our communication workshops, we frequently hear questions like these from experienced staff as well as new employees:

---

*Seers C. Talking to the elderly and its relavance to care. Nurs Times 1986;82:51.

- "Why does she keep asking me the same question?"
- "What does he mean he wants his mother? I've told him over and over, she's dead!"
- "Why can't I talk her into taking her bath?"
- "What do I say when he accuses me of taking his wallet?"
- "How can I get her to stop yelling all the time?"

A fourth goal of this handbook is to explore sensitive communication issues that affect everyone in today's institutions. One of these issues is cultural diversity. Multicultural hiring is a growing reality in the nursing home industry. Yet to date, institutions have done little to adopt programs or practices that soften the impact of diversity on staff and residents.

Another explosive issue is the verbal abuse and communication neglect of residents. Newspapers and television programs are filled with stories about residents who suffer abuse from professional caregivers. At the same time, direct care staff tell numerous tales of patients abusing caregivers. Research and clinical experience reveal the importance of effective communication in crisis prevention and in the restoration of order. Yet the role of communication in these circumstances is seldom the subject of in-service training and can rarely be found in orientation manuals for new employees. *Successful Communication with Alzheimer's Disease Patients* encourages candid discussion about verbal abuse and reminds the reader of the constant need for intercultural and intergenerational understanding, empathy, and patience.

An equally important issue is the communication problems and impairments of the caregivers themselves. Like cultural differences and verbal abuse, the personal communication shortcomings of caregivers are seldom addressed in a work setting where employees are surrounded by residents who have "real" problems. Caregivers must be open to each of these three issues if their Alzheimer's disease patients are going to receive optimum care.

A fifth and final goal of *Successful Communication with Alzheimer's Disease Patients* is to encourage administrators to establish high standards and set long-range policies that support effective communication throughout the facility. Time and money are interdependent resources. Both of these assets are protected when intelligent communication practices are at the center of every procedure.

The communication skills involved in giving clear instructions, listening actively, and detecting subtle signs of trouble in patients whose speech is disordered are basic to accident prevention. A staff trained to place high priority on effective communication makes fewer mistakes, has fewer accidents, and improves the safety record of the nursing home.

In addition, good communication promotes higher levels of worker satisfaction, which in turn results in lower absenteeism and employee turnover, which have a direct impact on budgets. An institution is at risk for losing important financial support when, on a regular basis, there are not enough people on shift to do an adequate job or to properly complete records. Staff time spent in rehiring and retraining new employees is always costly. The cost of continuing education programs in communication is cheap by comparison.

Good communication policies also improve the public image of an institution. The reputation of any organization is closely related to how management chooses to communicate about the institution to the local community. Research has shown that residents are more content when caregivers know how to use positive communication techniques to coax rather than to use constraints, coercion, or neglect. When residents are content, families are more easily reassured that they have made the correct placement decision.

Winning favor in the eyes of the local community is also an excellent way to raise the number of quality job applicants and build a solid volunteer work force. An astute administration will publicize innovative programs for the residents and publicly reward any educational or on-the-job achievements of its employees, especially the direct care staff.

In summary, the goals of this handbook are

1. To make the job of working with Alzheimer's disease residents easier, more efficient, and more pleasant.
2. To provide the highest quality of life available to the Alzheimer's disease resident.
3. To furnish all nursing home employees with basic information on communication processes, problems, and strengths of the Alzheimer's disease patient.
4. To promote discussion and problem-solving related to sensitive communication issues.
5. To encourage administrators and managers to design policies and procedures that support facility-wide use of effective communication.

OVERVIEW OF *SUCCESSFUL COMMUNICATION WITH ALZHEIMER'S DISEASE PATIENTS*

1. *Design: Successful Communication with Alzheimer's Disease Patients* is designed as a series of "how-to," in-service programs.

The intent has been to develop materials that are understandable, whether the reader has the support of a course structure or is using the text for independent study. Convenient features include:

- Quick tip summaries of key information
- Text outlines at the beginning of each unit
- Real-life examples, case studies, and scripts from actual encounters with Alzheimer's disease patients
- Self-study questionnaires, checklists, and quizzes
- Suggestions for team or group discussions, role plays, and activities
- Overheads of all quick tip summaries and definitions

2. *Structure:* Unit 1 of *Successful Communication with Alzheimer's Disease Patients* provides the student with a frame of reference—why and how we communicate, and what the various aspects of communication are. Units 2 and 3 describe the common communication disorders of Alzheimer's disease patients. Students learn that while many difficulties relate directly to the disease, other communication impairments are the result of aging, illness, and psychosocial factors. Units 4 and 5, perhaps the most practical units in the handbook, discuss how physical and psychosocial environments impact on the Alzheimer's disease resident's ability to communicate. The theme of these units is that even a small change in these environments can make a big difference in a patient's responsiveness.

Unit 6 addresses a very important yet little acknowledged issue—that of the professional caregiver's own communication strengths and weaknesses. This unit underscores the caregiver's responsibility in the communication process and contains many suggestions for helping caregivers care for themselves. Units 7 and 8 examine caregivers' communication styles, giving special attention to cultural diversity and verbal abuse. Open discussion of these sensitive issues is encouraged.

In Units 9 and 10, students learn specific communication techniques for enhancing conversation with Alzheimer's disease patients, and for using communication to prevent or limit troublesome situations. Within these two units caregivers will find the real "how-to" of communicating successfully with Alzheimer's disease patients.

Unit 11 encourages direct care staff to see the resident's family and friends as powerful resources, especially in communication. No one knows better what the patient likes and dislikes than the primary family caregiver. This information can save valuable time in situations that require the patient's cooperation. Unit 12 describes several formal programs or methods designed to support communication skills in patients with dementia. The programs have been successfully research-tested within the nursing home setting.

Of course, we realize that not all problems in a nursing home can be solved solely by improving or supporting the communication skills of residents and staff. Nevertheless, mastery of the concepts and skills contained in *Successful Communication with Alzheimer's Disease Patients* will help caregivers discover more situations that can be managed better, and with less effort, than they might ever have imagined. Good luck!

MJSP
EO

Introduction

The next few pages contain many suggestions for making the best use of *Successful Communication with Alzheimer's Disease Patients*. These include guidelines for instructor qualifications; possible sequences of presentation of units; ideas for attracting students; detailed lists for implementing smooth-running and successful programs; and recommendations for achieving maximum teaching effectiveness.

SELECTING AN INSTRUCTOR

A major presenting symptom of Alzheimer's disease is a decline in communication skills. One of the ways caregivers can most effectively manage Alzheimer's disease patients is through the use of facilitative communication techniques. *Successful Communication with Alzheimer's Disease Patients* is designed to provide a basis for in-service training in facilitative communication techniques.

Because of the close relationship between the disease process, communication skills, and the management of Alzheimer's disease patients, a speech-language pathologist is the ideal choice for instructor, consultant, or co-planner of a series of in-service communication training sessions.

Much of the significant research on the language and speech characteristics of aging and persons with dementia has been carried out by speech-language pathologists. These professionals receive rigorous training in diagnosis, treatment, and counseling of persons who have communication and swallowing disorders. Speech-language pathologists who work in nursing homes, home health care settings, and adult day-care centers specialize in the gerontologic aspects of communication and are experienced in providing in-service training programs. Their national professional organization, the American Speech-Language-Hearing Association, is a rich resource for additional materials on communication problems associated with aging and dementia.

Training can also be conducted by other health care professionals or the director of in-service training for the facility. The instructor should be well versed in the theory of adult education and possess superior interactive skills. This person should have a thorough understanding of the language changes that occur in residents with Alzheimer's disease and be skillful in responding to them. Finally, the instructor should be prepared to set aside ample time to prepare for each class and to collect follow-up data.

OPTIONS FOR PRESENTATION OF IN-SERVICE TRAINING UNITS

In-service training sessions may be taught

1. *Based on the sequence in this manual.* This manual has three sections and 12 units. The instructor may choose to present the units in the order in which they appear. The material is arranged so that background information on the communication problems of Alzheimer's disease patients appears in Part I; special concerns about caregivers' communication styles are presented in Part II; and suggestions, solutions, and specific techniques for improving communication in nursing homes are introduced in Part III. The units can be offered at regular intervals, such as one unit per month, or as a workshop over 2 or 3 days. When the units are taught in sequence, the knowledge and skills of the students build over time. The group of students in the ongoing class becomes a corps of communication specialists who can share their knowledge with other staff.

2. *Based on the special needs of the nursing home.* An instructor may not have the time, location, sufficient staff, or administrative support to present all 12 units in order. Therefore, the content, overheads, tests, and activities have been arranged so that any unit can be presented as a single in-service session. The instructor might wish to assign background reading from earlier units to prospective students so that they come into class with a basic understanding of communication and of Alzheimer's disease.

To properly select an in-service training unit, the training director should conduct a needs assessment. Invaluable data can be found in surveys of direct care staff, accident and catastrophic incident reports, occurrences of abuse, complaints from family members, personnel records on absenteeism and turnover, and exit interviews of employees who are leaving their jobs.[1] Do not wait to select a unit for study until a situation is so bad that "something (anything will do) has to be done." Instruction in effective communication should not be a "Band-Aid" attempt at crisis intervention.

3. *As an independent study.* The organization of *Successful Communication with Alzheimer's Disease Patients* is ideal for independent study. The format of this manual provides many opportunities for

students to review and test their own knowledge. In settings where opportunities for continuing education are few, independent study may be the only option. Independent study also works well for persons who must make up a missed class in order to obtain credit for completing all 12 units.

A major disadvantage to independent study is that students miss group discussions, problem solving, and role plays. Peer learning is a powerful benefit of group interaction. Students acquire knowledge through reading and lectures, but they are able to make more substantial behavioral changes when they participate actively.

4. *As an in-depth study of a single aspect of communication.* *Successful Communication with Alzheimer's Disease Patients* offers supervisors and program directors many ideas for conducting audits. For example, an audit might examine individual communication styles as described in Unit 6 and result in programs to help caregivers become better communicators. Environmental concerns, such as those presented in Units 4 and 5, could be ideal starting points in the on-going search for inexpensive ways to improve communication conditions in nursing homes. Although communication audits take staff time and energy, the nursing home that seeks to achieve superior status among peers cannot long overlook their long-term benefits.[2]

ENSURING THE SUCCESS OF IN-SERVICE TRAINING SESSIONS

Successful in-service training sessions may be ensured by

1. *Promoting participation.* Why do staff members attend an in-service training session? They may have negative incentives such as the need to meet mandatory regulations, to keep from being fired, or to get out of work temporarily. But staff members might also have positive reasons for attending training sessions on communication and Alzheimer's disease. Perhaps they are looking for a promotion, a pay raise, or a coveted certification. Perhaps completion offers them greater status in the eyes of their peers and the community. Best of all, perhaps they see the in-service training as a means of improving their own job satisfaction and the quality of care they provide their patients. The point is, training directors will have less trouble recruiting and persuading staff to stay with the program if they emphasize the potential benefits. Here are several suggestions for providing and promoting benefits:

    a. Develop an in-house certification program for employees who complete all 12 units. Use the certificate program as a starting point for implementing one or several of the following ideas.

b. Link the certificate or the completion of a certain number of communication in-service training sessions to promotions and pay raises.

c. Arrange with the state or corporate office for attendees to receive continuing education credit. This book contains outlines, quizzes, and quick tip summaries in ready-to-go formats and should supply ample evidence to reviewers that the course is worthy of continuing education credits.

d. Invent a title and new responsibilities for persons who have finished all 12 units of the manual (e.g., communication specialist). Such persons would assist with additional in-service training sessions, conduct audits or long-term studies, recruit new participants, write articles on communication for the in-house newsletter, or have responsibility for contacting the community press to publicize the program.

e. Create incentives that motivate students to finish the program and that also teach behavioral change: design a monthly competition prize for the person who makes more frequent use of one of the conversational strategies; who spots the highest number of physical barriers to communication; who writes the most detailed description of a patient's communication skills and deficits. Midway through the program, arrange a mini-celebration, a small reward, or some type of recognition, e.g., a "half-way" certificate; 2 hours of compensatory time; an empty frame for the anticipated certificate of completion; a bookmark inscribed with an inspirational quotation; an article for the in-house newsletter that mentions each student's name; one day's parking privilege in the chief executive officer's parking place; a letter to each attendee's supervisor with copies for each personnel file or a flower or special ribbon to be worn that day (others will ask about the significance of the flower or ribbon, which adds visibility to the program).

f. Keep the students' interest high by offering a variety of channels for information and experience during the sessions. Arrange a visit to the local university's speech and hearing clinic. Contract with an audiologist to screen each student's hearing and to speak briefly about the effects of hearing loss on job performance. Ask a lawyer to explain state laws and regulations regarding elder abuse and the "whistle-blower" protection clauses for persons who report suspected abusive acts. Invite a foreign-born staff member or volunteer to talk about the cultural differences in communication that he or she has observed since arriving in the United States.

g. Emphasize management's commitment to improving the communication climate in the nursing home by arranging for one of the top administrators to drop in and meet each student personally. This individual should be someone who knows about and strongly supports the program.

h. Extend the teaching and learning power of the in-service sessions by assigning pairs of students to give 10- or 15-minute mini-seminars on their own units. Ask them to review their experiences during the next communication in-service session. Students will have a firmer grasp of material that they have taught to others; feedback from their audiences and their class peers will solidify the learning.

i. Invite a local newspaper photographer to the graduation of staff members who have completed the entire series of communication units. Have a press release ready with the names and hometowns of all participants. Make sure that all names are spelled correctly.

j. Cultivate new or future students by offering recruitment incentives similar to the suggestions offered in (d) above. Toward the end of an in-service training series, ask the students to speak with and recommend prospective participants for the next series.

k. Advertise the program to the volunteer corps as well as to staff members. Encourage, or better yet, require the participation of volunteers in at least one in-service session on communication or make participation a routine part of new volunteer orientation. Include the opportunity for communication training in all nursing home literature that recruits volunteers.

l. Cut costs by co-sponsoring the program with the training department of another nearby nursing home or the local college or home health agency that conducts nursing assistant certification programs.

2. *Paying attention to details of preparation.* Nursing homes with well-established training departments usually have a set of checklists and procedures for making logistical arrangements before an in-service training program. In-service training planners working in institutions with little or no pre-training organizational aids will need to create a list and a set of timelines for keeping track of details. The use of these checklists reduces distractions and crises during the sessions, supports a higher quality of instruction, and keeps students coming back. Items to include on the checklist are:

a. Conduct a needs assessment to determine the starting point of the program.
b. Obtain administrative approval.
c. Initiate the continuing education unit (CEU) or certification approval process.
d. Contract with an instructor or instructors, or make site arrangements for the field trip.
e. Enlist the aid of an in-service training assistant. This person's mission is to share in the preparation and follow-up of the program, to make the instructor's job as stress-free as possible, and to arrange an ideal environment for learning.
f. Schedule the room.
g. Determine the need for and reserve audiovisual equipment.
h. Circulate announcements of the program.
j. Make arrangements for taking reservations from prospective students.
k. Arrange for refreshments if desired.
l. Assemble and copy handouts.
m. Assemble and copy course evaluation sheets, notices to floor supervisors if necessary, certificates of completion, CEU credit forms, and letters for personnel files.
n. Decide on and assemble materials for incentives.
o. Check to see if the audiovisual equipment works and if the instructor knows how to operate it. Have an extra light bulb for the overhead projector available.
p. Make sure there are enough desks or tables and chairs, trash cans, chalk or markers and erasers, toilet paper in the bathrooms, etc.
q. For the last session: Ask the publicity or marketing department to schedule a photographer and to have an article written for the in-house newsletter and the community press. Invite a special guest to present certificates of completion.
r. Record and analyze immediate post-training evaluation sheets for program improvement.
s. Conduct follow-up assessments, such as interviews or surveys with the supervisors or students. Analyze results to see if the students' behaviors have improved.
t. Present final data analysis to the administration to justify program continuation or expansion.
u. Publicize results through the in-house newsletter, the local newspaper, regional or national professional journals, or professional conventions and seminars.

3. *Encouraging creative teaching styles.* The object of offering in-service training to employees is not just to change their level of knowledge but also to change their behavior. For behavioral changes to occur, the class structure must offer students numerous opportunities to actively work on their behaviors. Therefore, students should be expected to read the text of a unit before coming to class. With only 60 minutes available, instructors could limit lectures to 15–20 minutes and fill the remaining time with practical activities. Some examples would be brainstorming for solutions to real problems faced by the participants, sharing case studies and personal experiences, probing into the theory and ethics that underlie the institution's communication policies, setting up assignments for students to teach the material to others, assessing skills and attitudes, and role playing to try new methods and gain new insights. "Solely presenting knowledge about a topic [through lectures] is an ineffectual method for changing staff behaviors."[3]

Instructors should be skillful in establishing a comfortable environment for discussion of "taboo" subjects and sensitive issues. The instructor is responsible for setting an example of trust and confidentiality for the group. Students also need to feel safe when trying new techniques. Although role playing is supposed to be one of the best forms of teaching and learning,[4] some people are uncomfortable performing in front of their peers. No one likes the feeling that the people with whom they work might laugh at them if they do something "stupid" or "wrong." The instructor must realize that the trust and fun that emerge from good role playing build gradually as a group bonds together during repeated sessions. One suggestion for breaking the "performance ice" is to introduce a short game of charades, using the nursing home's slogans, situations, and procedures as material. Another is to have two students read aloud from sample scripts, such as those that appear at the end of Unit 9. One person takes the part of the caregiver, another the patient.

Below are more guidelines for conducting successful role plays, adapted from Coury and Lubinski's chapter in *Dementia and Communication*[4]:

- Students should be encouraged to "think on their feet."
- Let the student play himself or herself while the instructor plays patient; then replay the problem situation and reverse roles.
- Stop the action if a player becomes too anxious or runs out of ideas.
- Ask the audience to make suggestions to help the player.

- Start the role play over to give players a second chance for a positive experience.
- Coach the players in coping with emotionally charged statements. For example, "You're frustrated, even angry by now. She hit you."
- Summarize strategies for communication repair frequently for the group. Ask them to judge which strategies would be most effective with particular patients with whom they work.
- Videotape the role play to capture fine teaching points and illustrate good use of technique, but only after students have had some practice with role playing.

REFERENCES

1. MacNamara R. Lessons from Human Service Administration in Organized Care Settings for the Elderly and Handicapped. Springfield, IL: Thomas, 1988.
2. Tellis-Nayak V. Nursing Home Exemplars of Quality: The Paths to Excellence in Quality Nursing Homes. Springfield, IL: Thomas, 1988.
3. Lubinski R. Dementia and Communication. Philadelphia: BC Decker, 1991;286.
4. Coury LN, Lubinsky R. Effective In-Service Training for Staff Working With Communication Impaired Patients. In R Lubinsky (ed), Dementia and Communication. Philadelphia: BC Decker, 1991;279.

PART I

Alzheimer's Disease Patients and Their Environment

UNIT
1

Communication in the Nursing Home

UNIT OUTLINE

Premise
1. We depend on communication to accomplish most of life's tasks.
2. Effective communication promotes understanding and a sense of well-being in patients and staff.

Definitions
Communication
Effective Communication
Communication Competence
Verbal Communication
Nonverbal Communication
Quick Tip Summary: Nonverbal Communication

Why We Communicate
Quick Tip Summary: Why We Communicate

Why Effective Communication in a Nursing Home is so Important
Quick Tip Summary: Importance of Effective Communication in the Nursing Home

Requirements for Effective Communication
1. A place
2. A shared language
3. A common frame of reference
4. A certain set of mental abilities
5. Openness
6. Expectation of response
7. Respect and trust
Quick Tip Summary: Requirements for Effective Communication

Some Final Notes on Communication

References

PREMISE

We depend on communication to accomplish most of life's tasks. The better we communicate, the more likely that we will be understood and will get what we need from other people. When we do not communicate effectively, misunderstandings develop and mistakes are made. In a nursing home, effective communication not only ensures accurate decision-making and efficiency, but also promotes understanding and a sense of well-being in residents and staff members.

DEFINITIONS

Communication

Communication occurs when a person sends or receives messages and when meaning is assigned to another person's signals. Every act of communication takes place in a specific *environment* that has *physical* and *psychosocial* aspects. Each person involved in communication is both a *source* (speaker) and a *receiver* (listener).

Spoken words provide as little as 7% of any message communicated between two people. *Expression,* or how the words are said (e.g., sadly or sarcastically), accounts for 35% of any message communicated, and *body language* accounts for approximately 58% of any message.[1] This means that as much as 93% of our messages are communicated nonverbally.

Human beings are always communicating. In fact, when two people are in the same room, it is impossible for them *not* to communicate. Because communication is 58% body language, messages are sent even when no words are said. Lovers, enemies, competitors, casual acquaintances, and complete strangers convey volumes to one another without ever saying a word. We humans may not always communicate intentionally or effectively, but we are always communicating *something* to *someone.*

Effective Communication

A message is communicated effectively when its intent is accurately understood by another, who then responds appropriately.

Communication Competence
The ability to communicate effectively is called *communication competence*. Simply stated, the greater a person's knowledge of communication, the greater his or her communication competence. The more ways you have to express yourself, the greater the likelihood you will communicate effectively in any situation.

Verbal Communication
The actual words spoken constitute verbal communication. (See also definitions of "Speech," "Language," and "Voice," in Unit 3.)

Nonverbal Communication
Nonverbal signals constitute as much as 93% of any message. Culture, personality, and emotions contribute to an individual's style of nonverbal communication. These nonverbal signals include:

- Expression—the rate of speaking and the pitch, volume, and intonation of the voice
- Body position—proximity to the listener; at eye level, above, or below the listener
- Body orientation—positioning toward or away from the listener
- Gesture—the presence, frequency, and expressiveness of hand and body movements
- Touch—the presence, meaningfulness, and gentleness of touch
- Facial expression and eye contact—the ability to show interest, emotion, and empathy
- Personal appearance—the condition of clothes, hairstyle, cosmetics, and scents
- Personal environment—choices of living quarters, music, and companions

Nonverbal communication serves many purposes. It can emphasize or repeat what is said verbally. It can substitute for verbal communication, as when the speaker shrugs his or her shoulders rather than admit, "I don't know." Nonverbal communication can regulate verbal communication. If you lower your voice at the end of a sentence, you are letting your conversational partner know your turn is over. When you turn away from someone, you are rejecting further conversation. Sometimes, too, nonverbal communication contradicts verbal communication, as when a person with a red face and bulging veins yells, "Angry? No, I am not angry!"

Nonverbal styles vary from person to person. Some people use nonverbal signals generously to enhance their communication.

A script writer once complained to movie producer Sam Goldwyn, "I'm telling you a sensational story. All I'm asking for is your opinion, and you fall asleep!" Mr. Goldwyn responded, "Isn't sleeping an opinion?"

Illustration 1.1   Nonverbal Communication

Others rarely use gestures and facial expression. Sometimes we send unintentional messages because we are not aware of the nonverbal signals we have used. Remember, we cannot *not* communicate (Illustration 1.1).

Sharpen your awareness of the nonverbal messages you are sending. Also, develop an awareness of the nonverbal messages that Alzheimer's disease patients send when they do not have the words to speak or when their words do not convey how they really feel.

Quick Tip Summary: Nonverbal Communication

1. We are always communicating. Most of the information we communicate is transmitted nonverbally.
2. Nonverbal communication can augment, repeat, or substitute for verbal information. It can also control or contradict verbal communication. Nonverbal communication often reveals our true feelings.
3. The amount and type of nonverbal communication we use and understand is determined by our cultures, our families, and our personalities.
4. Some people use nonverbal communication more effectively than others.
5. The ability to use and interpret nonverbal communication helps us work more effectively with Alzheimer's disease patients.

WHY WE COMMUNICATE

We have defined communication as the sending and receiving of messages, but communication is more than the exchange of information between people. The most important reason that people communicate is to meet their individual needs. We communicate with people who can help us obtain necessities, such as food, shelter, and clothing. Communication helps us secure our safety and protects us from danger, whether it is calling the police or reading a "Slippery When Wet" sign.

Communication is also essential to the fulfillment of our most basic social and emotional needs. Others can only show love, acceptance, and concern for us through communication. When we do not receive expressions of love and acceptance, we are at risk for major health problems—depression, failure-to-thrive syndrome, heart disease, and cancer to name just a few.

Communication meets our need for self-actualization. By communicating, we let other people know who we are, what we are doing, and the principles on which we stand. Without communication, we would have no professional, political, or educational expression.

Another reason we communicate is to exert power or control over other people. Communication is our chief means of managing others, of trying to get others to do what we want. Finally, we use communication to meet the needs of others—to provide them with information, praise, and support and to express our affection for them. We care for others through our words and gestures. Communication is a powerful therapeutic tool. Through communication, we help restore psychological well-being to others and to ourselves.

Quick Tip Summary: Why We Communicate[2]
We communicate:

1. To give and gain information.
2. To meet our need for food, shelter, and clothing; security and safety.
3. To meet our need for social and emotional health.
4. To engage in self-actualization and self-disclosure.
5. To control, exert power, and manage.
6. To meet the needs of others.
7. As a therapeutic tool.

WHY EFFECTIVE COMMUNICATION IN A NURSING HOME IS SO IMPORTANT

When people communicate effectively, they achieve more of their goals and have more satisfaction in their lives. In a nursing home, effective communication is especially important. Effective communication saves time. If people understand a message the first time, the communicator does not have to waste time repeating it. Effective communication prevents mistakes. If people understand instructions, they are less likely to make mistakes that must be remedied later.

Effective communication has a beneficial effect on nursing home residents and caregivers alike. It reduces power struggles, calms patients, and prevents catastrophic behaviors. In return, caregivers experience less stress, and there is less potential for abusive incidents. Effective communication provides the caregiver with critical information about the patient. If a caregiver knows the capabilities of a patient, the caregiver can allow that person to do more and thereby prevent a build-up of learned helplessness. (See definition of "Learned Helplessness" in Unit 2.)

Effective communication reduces the isolation and depersonalization of patients and caregivers. Sharing each other's accomplishments, problems, backgrounds, likes, and dislikes builds self-esteem and promotes personal bonding between caregivers and patients.

From an administrative viewpoint, effective communication can clearly reduce the level of worker stress and reduce the rate of worker burnout. The bottom line is that effective communication in a nursing home can and does save the facility money.

Quick Tip Summary: Importance of Effective Communication in a Nursing Home
Effective communication:

1. Saves time.
2. Prevents mistakes; saves work later on.
3. Calms the patients; calms the caregivers.
4. Defuses power struggles; prevents catastrophic behaviors; reduces the potential for abusive incidents.
5. Prevents patients from learning helplessness.
6. Reduces isolation and depersonalization of patients and caregivers.
7. Promotes personal bonding between patients and caregivers.
8. Promotes self-esteem in patients and caregivers.
9. Cuts down on worker stress; reduces high rates of caregiver burnout.
10. Saves money for the facility.

REQUIREMENTS FOR EFFECTIVE COMMUNICATION

Think of the last time you had a real heart-to-heart conversation with a close friend or loved one. A heart-to-heart conversation is one of the best illustrations of effective communication. What does it take to make a heart-to-heart conversation work? What conditions are necessary?

1. *A place.* You need a place that is *quiet* and free of distractions; a place that is *private* and *comfortable*. Quiet, private, comfortable places are difficult to find in many nursing homes.
2. *A shared language.* To have a heart-to-heart conversation, you and your friend must speak the same language. The less language you share, the tougher it is to communicate. Not only words, but also the body language of nods, gestures, and gaze can have dif-

ferent meanings in different languages. Even persons who speak different dialects of the same language can have different vocabularies. Gaps between the sexes and generations within each language also create communication breakdowns between people.

Seldom do residents and caregivers in a nursing home share a totally common language. They must often overcome regional, cultural, gender-related, and age-related differences to make communication work.

3. *A common frame of reference.* Every individual has a personal frame of reference, a personal set of experiences, interests, values, and beliefs. A frame of reference grows out of personal preference and experience, socioeconomic and cultural factors, and historical events. Persons who did not live through the Great Depression might not put as much value on job security as those who did. Persons who have never experienced persecution or prejudice may not be sensitive to the pain that particular words can cause Holocaust survivors or those who struggled through the civil rights movement. The people with whom you communicate best, with whom you like to have heart-to-heart conversations, generally share your frame of reference. Few workers in nursing homes truly share common frames of reference with the residents for whom they care, and vice versa.

4. *A certain set of mental abilities.* Certain basic mental abilities are required for effective communication. These include:

    a. *Perception.* To understand and respond to someone's message, two people must be able to see and hear each other. When having a heart-to-heart conversation, you tend to watch your partner's face and listen carefully. Many elderly nursing home residents have deficits in hearing and vision that interfere with their perception. Many caregivers, busy with their chores, do not look at residents while talking to them or do not listen to what the residents say. Important messages often go unnoticed.

    b. *Attention.* To communicate well, the speaker and the listener must be able to pay attention to each other. You do not feel like sharing your innermost feelings unless you have someone's close attention. One symptom of Alzheimer's disease and other dementias is difficulty in maintaining attention. Medications and anxieties also interfere with the ability to attend. Nursing home personnel are frequently too busy or distracted to pay close attention to residents' attempts at communication. Both partners miss messages because of lack of attention.

    c. *Intellectual understanding.* To communicate effectively, two people must be able to understand each other's ideas. You are unlikely to bother explaining your thoughts to persons who cannot grasp them. Alzheimer's disease robs people of the intellectual ability to understand. Caregivers, in turn, make fewer efforts to share information. The less intellectual stimulation the patients receive, the less practice they get in processing it. The inevitable decline in intellectual functioning is hastened by the lack of effective communication. An ongoing spiral of deterioration is set in motion.

d. *Memory.* To stay on topic and to add details to a story, a speaker must have adequate memory. *Long-term memory* is needed to remember the person with whom you are talking and the subject being discussed. *Short-term memory* is needed to remember your partner's questions and remarks long enough to form responses. Alzheimer's disease is characterized by the loss of memory. Caregivers, too, find that they cannot remember the details in the lives and medical histories of all the patients in their care. Limitations in the memories of patients and caregivers not only reduce the effectiveness of communication but also stifle the desire of either party to communicate.

5. *Openness.* Openness is a willingness to listen to and honestly appraise your partner's message even if you think you will not agree. If your partner is not open to your message, you are apt to withhold your ideas and opinions; you do not speak up if you think your words will "fall on deaf ears." Alzheimer's disease patients often appear self-absorbed and uninterested in the messages of others. Equally damaging to the communication process, however, are staff members who show little openness to the messages of residents. Many caregivers admit they have little desire to hear them.

6. *Expectation of response.* When you speak earnestly to someone, you expect a response—preferably a carefully worded answer, but at least a nonverbal acknowledgment! If your heart-to-heart partner were to sit silently after hearing your important announcement, you would probably say, "Well? Say something!" Research shows that patients with Alzheimer's disease continue to expect responses, too, until quite late in the illness. Their expectations often go unmet. Conversely, staff members seldom expect responses from these patients. They hurry on without realizing that low expectations beget low results.

7. *Respect and trust.* The final requirements for good communication are respect and trust. The person with whom you had your last heart-to-heart conversation was undoubtedly someone you respected and trusted. Otherwise you would not have told your secrets, shared your opinions, or bared your soul. You would not have felt safe.

New residents with Alzheimer's disease may find it hard to trust people in the unfamiliar setting of a nursing home. In nursing homes where the staff turnover rate is high, the formation of trusting relationships is especially difficult. Alzheimer's disease patients are often deeply suspicious of those who care for them. For their part, some caregivers appear not to respect the integrity of demented patients. They take for granted their right to enter a resident's room, search through belongings, and forcibly direct the patient's life. Some of these actions may be necessary, but their abrupt execution does not convey a sense of respect and trust; it engenders suspicion and defensiveness.

Quick Tip Summary: Requirements for Effective Communication
Effective communication requires:

1. A place.
2. A shared language.
3. A common frame of reference.
4. A certain set of mental abilities.
   a. Perception
   b. Attention
   c. Intellectual understanding
   d. Memory
5. Openness.
6. Expectation of response.
7. Respect and trust.

SOME FINAL NOTES ON COMMUNICATION

1. Effective communication is possible without one or more of the requirements discussed here. Lovers get engaged in a crowded subway, blind and deafened individuals manage businesses, and people from different cultures develop close friendships. However, the fewer requirements that can be met, the greater the effort communication partners must make in order to compensate. Learning to communicate effectively under less than optimal conditions is the greatest challenge faced by caregivers of Alzheimer's disease patients.

2. We tend to understand others based on our personal points of view and cultural biases. Everyone does.

3. Effective communication does not guarantee agreement. A good fight can still be good communication.

4. Our attitudes, or what we say to ourselves inside our heads, eventually find expression in how we behave and talk to others. A caregiver who thinks, "If he does that one more time, I'll. . . ." is more likely to speak with open irritation to that patient than a caregiver who thinks, "I'm going to stay calm when Joe starts insulting me again."

5. The only person we can control is ourselves. No one else can make us say anything we do not want to say. No one else can make us lose control over our actions if we know clearly what we are supposed to do.

6. We can change the ways we communicate. We can change our attitudes. With practice and experience, we can develop effective communication skills even though our Alzheimer's disease patients are losing theirs. This book is dedicated to the proposition that work with Alzheimer's disease patients can be improved tremendously by changing the ways *we* communicate.

REFERENCES

1. DeVito JA. Essentials of Human Communication. New York: HarperCollins, 1993;6.
2. R Lubinski (ed). Dementia and Communication. Philadelphia: BC Decker, 1991;142.

GOOD PRACTICE 1.1   BENEFITS OF GOOD COMMUNICATION

A. *Directions:* Write the corresponding number from the list in the section "Quick Tip Summary: The Importance of Effective Communication in a Nursing Home" for the examples below. If this activity is done as a group, discuss your answers together. Opinions may differ.

1. (   ) We don't have to cover for each other's absences on our unit now like we used to. I'm feeling less stressed, more like I can do my job as it should be done.
2. (   ) Last week we spent a total of one-half employee hour each day in social contact with one of our most combative residents (5-minute segments throughout the day and evening). His catastrophic reactions have dropped from two per day to three per week. (See definition of "Catastrophic Reaction" in Unit 10.)
3. (   ) Two of the residents with Alzheimer's disease on our unit are starting to feed themselves.
4. (   ) We have a new chart on our bulletin board. We select one resident with Alzheimer's disease each week. The staff member who can coax the highest number of responses from that resident (verbal or nonverbal) wins a lottery ticket.
5. (   ) Our supervisor provided us with 10 hours of communication training last year. It was useful at home and on the job. I wasn't surprised to learn that our unit now has the lowest rate of staff turnover in the facility.

B. *Directions:* In a team discussion, ask participants to describe their own real-life experiences related to the following benefits of good communication. In the spaces below, write the best example of each.

1. Saves time: _____

2. Prevents mistakes and accidents: _____

3. Calms the resident; calms the caregiver: _____

4. Reduces isolation of the caregiver and resident; promotes personal bonding: _____

5. Saves facility time and money: _____

Discussion Point: In what ways could these ideas be adapted to your unit or department?

GOOD PRACTICE 1.2   TUNING IN TO VERBAL AND NONVERBAL COMMUNICATION: A TELEVISION-BASED EXERCISE

Directions: Tune in to a popular TV soap opera or dramatic presentation. Set the kitchen timer for 1 minute. Close your eyes. Listen, then write down the different emotions you *heard* when the actors spoke.

A. Verbal Communication: Expression

1. Which emotions did you recognize? _____
    _____

2. What changes in the actors' voices let you know that different emotions were being expressed? _____
    _____

    ___Spoke faster   ___Voice was high   ___Speech was louder
    ___Spoke slower   ___Voice was low   ___Speech was softer

3. What else did you notice about listening to the conversation with your eyes closed? _____
    _____

B. Nonverbal Communication: Body Language

Now for 1 minute, open your eyes but turn off the TV sound. Watch the actors' body language and facial expressions.

If an actor used any of the gestures or postures listed below, write a word in the blank that names the emotion you think the actor was trying to show:

Head shake_____	Head nod_____
Head droop_____	Chin up_____
Shoulders droop_____	Shoulders hunched_____
Shoulders "squared"_____	Hands clenched_____
Hands "fiddling"_____	Body forward_____
Body relaxed, "open"_____	Arms or legs crossed_____
Wide, rapid stride_____	Slow stride_____

GOOD PRACTICE 1.3   EXPERIENCING EFFECTIVE COMMUNICATION: A PERSONAL EXERCISE

Directions: Think of the last time you had a true heart-to-heart communication with another person. Identify the place and language of the communication and answer yes (Y) or no (N) to the 20 questions. Add up the number of "yes" responses and multiply by five to get a percentage score. If your communication was effective, your score should be 80% or better.

Place where heart-to-heart occurred: _____

Language spoken in the conversation: _____

1. Was the place quiet? ( )
2. Was the place private? ( )
3. Was the place comfortable? ( )
4. Was the conversation in your native language? ( )
5. Was the conversation in your communication partner's native language? ( )
6. Did you and your communication partner share a common cultural background? ( )
7. Did you and your communication partner have a similar frame of reference? ( )
8. Could your partner hear what you said? ( )
9. Did your partner pay attention to your message? ( )
10. Did he or she understand your message? ( )
11. Could he or she remember what you said? ( )
12. Could you understand the meaning of your partner's message? ( )
13. Was your partner "open" to your message? ( )
14. Were you open to your partner's message? ( )
15. Did your partner respond to your message? ( )
16. Did you respond to your partner's message? ( )
17. Did you trust your partner? ( )
18. Did your partner appear to trust you? ( )
19. Did you respect your partner? ( )
20. Did your partner respect your ideas? ( )

Number of yes (Y) responses × 5 = _____%
(% overall communication effectiveness)

Discussion Point: In contrast, think of the last time you attempted to have a conversation with one of your Alzheimer's disease patients. If you scored that conversation on this scale, how would it compare to the first?

UNIT 2

Communication Problems and Strengths of Patients with Alzheimer's Disease and Related Disorders

UNIT OUTLINE

Premise

1. In spite of increasing communication deficits, Alzheimer's disease patients retain many functional communication abilities.
2. Caregivers can capitalize on the remaining communication strengths of Alzheimer's disease patients to compensate for those communication abilities that are lost.

Definitions

Communication Disorder

Communication Breakdown

Learned Helplessness

Communication Breakdowns Caused by Alzheimer's Disease

Communication Losses Characteristic of Alzheimer's Disease

Communication Changes Characteristic of Alzheimer's Disease

1. Stereotypic language
2. Empty speech
3. Paraphasias
4. Violations of conversational rules
5. Windows of lucidity

Communication Breakdowns Caused by the Aging Process

1. Loss of independence
2. Loss of livelihood and social role
3. Loss of physical attractiveness and grooming skills
4. Loss of energy
5. Loss of family and friends
6. Loss of familiar environments
7. Loss of first-language partners

PREMISE

Alzheimer's disease causes a person's communication skills to deteriorate along a predictable course. Deterioration of memory, understanding, speech, language, and social skills takes a toll on a patient's ability to communicate effectively. While some skills are lost, other abilities undergo characteristic changes. In addition, Alzheimer's patients experience communication breakdowns secondary to the aging process.

To better understand the communication behaviors of persons with Alzheimer's disease, caregivers must think not only about what is lost and what is changed, however, but also about what is preserved. The capacity for storytelling, for instance, is indeed lost, but the ability to use good sentence structure remains intact until late in the disease. Some skills, such as word finding, weaken almost from the beginning. Yet with the right kind of verbal support, most Alzheimer's disease patients can be helped to think of the words they want long into the course of the illness.

DEFINITIONS

Communication Disorder

A communication disorder is a condition that interferes with a person's ability to be understood or to understand the communication of others. Speech that deviates so far from the speech of others that it calls attention to itself or causes distress for the listener or the speaker is also considered to be a communication disorder.[1]

Communication Breakdown

Communication breakdown occurs when a listener does not understand the words and/or the intent of the speaker's message. Breakdowns in communication can happen for many reasons. They happen every day to everyone and they are not always the result of a communication disorder.

Learned Helplessness

"Learned helplessness arises when persons learn through repeated experiences that their actions have little effect on the outcome of the situation—especially in the 'restricted' environment of a nursing home."[2]

COMMUNICATION BREAKDOWNS CAUSED BY ALZHEIMER'S DISEASE

As a patient goes from the early to the middle and late stages of Alzheimer's disease, the number of lost abilities increases and the changes become more marked.

Communication Losses Characteristic of Alzheimer's Disease

In Table 2.1, communication abilities are divided into four categories: *memory, understanding, speech and language skills*, and *social skills*. The table explains which abilities persons with Alzheimer's disease lose as their disease progresses.

Communication Changes Characteristic of Alzheimer's Disease

Professional caregivers will quickly recognize some characteristic changes that appear in the communication of Alzheimer's patients.

1. *Stereotypic language.* Persons with Alzheimer's disease use more stereotypic language in their everyday exchanges. They are apt to make remarks, such as "You got me!" or "Can't say as I do." or "Easier said than done!" over and over again.

2. *Empty speech.* Alzheimer's disease patients tend to talk in generalizations or empty speech. Specific words that tell the listener "who," "what," or "where" are replaced by more vague or general terms. Instead of saying, "Please warm up my coffee in the microwave on the counter," an Alzheimer's disease patient in the middle stages of the disease might say, "Here, put this in that thing over there."

3. *Paraphasias.* Alzheimer's disease patients frequently confuse words that are related. Sometimes they say the opposite of what

Table 2.1 Communication Losses Characteristic of Alzheimer's Disease

Stage	Memory	Understanding	Speech and language skills	Social skills
Early	Loses time orientation. Loses some long-term and short-term memory (not always apparent in conversation). Loses recently acquired information. Cannot retain five-item lists or phone numbers.	Loses ability to understand rapid speech, speech in noisy or distracting environment, complex or abstract conversation, sarcastic humor or innuendo.	Loses ideas of what to talk about. Loses ability to process language rapidly. Slow processing apparent in pauses and hesitancies. Loses rapid naming ability—uses related words such as "salt" for "sugar" (ability to self-correct retained).	Loses ability to stay on topic. Loses control over anger and argumentativeness. Loses "conversational bridges," making speech seem blunt and rude. Loses ability to pay attention to speaker for more than a few minutes.
Middle	Loses time and place orientation (not person). Loses additional long-term and short-term memory (apparent in conversation). Loses abstract vocabulary and concepts, names of less-familiar people. Cannot remember 3-item lists or 3-step commands. Cannot retain information shortly after presented.	Loses ability to understand ordinary, prolonged conversation. Loses ability to focus and maintain attention in presence of distraction or noise. Loses ability to understand what is read, although mechanics of reading are preserved. Loses some ability to read facial cues, although perception of emotional meaning is retained.	Loses naming abilities, especially abstract or specific words. Loses fluency: more pauses, revisions, and sentence fragments. Loses ability to self-correct. Loses loudness of voice and vocal expression in conversation. Loses creative, "original" use of language. Loses ability to finish sentences.	Cannot see things from another's point of view; becomes more egocentric. Asks fewer questions. Starts fewer conversations. Makes less eye contact. Seldom comments or self-corrects. Withdraws from social situations. Loses "niceness" in conversation.
Late	Loses orientation to time, place, and person. Loses ability to form new memories. Loses ability to recognize family members.	Loses ability to understand most word meanings. Loses overall awareness. Doesn't seem to know when being spoken to.	Loses grammar and diction; speaks in jargon. May lose speech altogether, may become mute.	Loses awareness of social interaction or expectations. Loses apparent desire to communicate.

Source: Adapted from E Ostuni, MJ Santo Pietro. Getting Through: Communicating When Someone You Care for Has Alzheimer's Disease. Vero Beach, FL: Speech Bin, 1991;12.

In addition to Alzheimer's disease, poor health was taking a toll on Grandma K. She was dying of pneumonia. She had not spoken in more than 6 months and did not appear to recognize anyone. Her daughter, Harriet, called all the grandchildren to the nursing home; Grandma K. was not expected to live through the night. The last to arrive was the youngest, John, who was in his late twenties. John raced down the hall, found Grandma K.'s room, and stood panting in the doorway. The entire family was assembled around the old woman's bed. Grandma K. opened one eye, looked directly at her grandson and said, "John, did you ever get married?"

Illustration 2.1   Window of Lucidity

they mean; sometimes they say a word that is wrong but comes from the same category (e.g., "hot" instead of "cold" or "salt" instead of "sugar"). These errors are called paraphasias.

4. *Violations of conversational rules.* Violations of conversational rules are statements or comments that break the unwritten rules of normal human conversation. They are responses that are inappropriate, egocentric, blunt, or rude. Crying, walking away, swearing, or making a totally unrelated statement are typical violations of conversational rules.

5. *Windows of lucidity.* A window of lucidity is a moment or two in time when an Alzheimer's disease patient suddenly remembers things or talks clearly about ideas that appeared to be long forgotten (Illustration 2.1). All Alzheimer's disease patients seem to experience occasional windows of lucidity.

COMMUNICATION BREAKDOWNS CAUSED BY THE AGING PROCESS

Most patients with Alzheimer's disease are old. Part of growing old is coming face-to-face with many losses, and these losses directly affect the ways in which people communicate. The communication disabilities of Alzheimer's disease patients are compounded by the losses they experience because of the aging process.

1. *Loss of independence.* Most elderly nursing home residents lose their physical and financial independence. The entire dynamic of their communication with others therefore changes. Their energy becomes consumed with getting through another day; all they seem to talk about are their physical ailments and the possessions they once had.

Marya was having a tough day. "Come on, sweetie," she cajoled Mr. Miller, "time to get dressed for breakfast. Gotta look nice for all the ladies!" Mr. Miller made no response. "Manny, did you hear me?" Still he made no response. Marya's patience ran short. "Hey, come on. This is the third time I've asked you this morning. Now you do what I say, Mister, or you'll be sorry!" (This was the same thing she had said to her 9-year-old that morning.) Suddenly Mr. Miller exploded, "Who do you think you are, telling me when to get dressed? I'll get dressed when I damned well please! Now get out of my room!"

Illustration 2.2   Parent-Child Power Struggle

Some caregivers find it hard to treat a person who is no longer physically independent as an equal. They talk to and treat dependent elderly residents as if they were children. Elderly residents, including those with Alzheimer's disease, typically respond to this "parent-child" attitude in one of two ways: either they settle comfortably into the dependent role and develop a crippling *learned helplessness* ("I can't do anything unless you help me"), or they react angrily and defensively (Illustration 2.2). Either way, communication that is based on a caregiver's parent-child attitude creates problems.

Financial dependence also generates communication problems for nursing home residents. Many patients do not have the resources to obtain essentials or simple pleasures. Long distance telephone calls, new bottles of cologne, or hearing-aid batteries must be handled or purchased by relatives or caregivers. The patient can only hope that others will remember his or her personal needs and preferences.

2. *Loss of livelihood and social role.* Most of us define ourselves by what we do for a living and by our place in the family and the community. How we talk to others is determined by the roles we play in jobs, families, and society. When we no longer have those roles, we lose our usual communication places and partners; our role-related vocabulary is no longer useful. For this reason, some elderly persons feel isolated despite the crowds in the nursing home. They feel that they have little in common with other residents, and, literally, that they are not who they once were. Knowing "who they used to be" is an important part of the role of the professional caregiver.

3. *Loss of physical attractiveness and grooming skills.* Loss of physical attractiveness presents a very real barrier to communication. Research has shown that people are more likely to choose "attractive" rather than "unattractive" persons for communication partners. Dry wrinkled skin, cloudy eyes, yellow toenails, and other changes to an aging body are not on most people's lists of "beautiful

Martha, an 81-year-old retired pharmacist, spent most of her days alone in her room. The unit staff members were concerned because, although she was still capable, she was speaking less and less to others. One of the nurse's aides brought Martha the news that Mr. Simms, a long-time pharmacist from a local drugstore, had recently entered the home. Perhaps, the aide suggested enthusiastically, Martha and Mr. Simms would enjoy sitting together for lunch once in a while. "You could talk about your pharmacies," the aide offered. "What?" scoffed Martha, "That old man?"

Illustration 2.3   Perception of Old as Unattractive

features." Senior citizens are no different from most people. They, too, shun what they perceive as "unattractive" (Illustration 2.3).

Loss of physical attractiveness is made worse by the effects of the deteriorating grooming skills of patients with Alzheimer's disease. Unkempt hair, body odor, the smell of urine or halitosis, unshaven stubble, all these discourage potential communication partners. Furthermore, people who feel disheveled often do not feel like socializing. It is especially crucial to keep residents with Alzheimer's disease looking and smelling good. They become progressively less aware of their grooming as they become more impaired in their communication. The grooming process itself can be an excellent opportunity for communication between patient and caregiver. There are good memories associated with being pampered and made beautiful. A resident with Alzheimer's disease who senses that he or she is well groomed may feel more like seeking companionship or at least like accepting the approach of others more readily.

4. *Loss of energy.* When energy levels are low, people feel less like making an effort to talk. All elderly people experience some loss of vigor as a normal part of the aging process. Institutionalized elderly persons get little exercise, little time outdoors, and diminished intellectual and emotional stimulation, all of which result in a major loss of energy, even before medications and pureed diets are introduced. Activities, foods, and sensory stimulation that increase energy levels will have a direct impact on the motivation of an Alzheimer's disease patient to communicate.

5. *Loss of family and friends.* It is a fact of life that as a person gets older, more and more loved ones disappear. The people with whom that person has been communicating most intimately—parents, siblings, spouses, coworkers, and friends—pass away or move away or visit the nursing home less often. These losses are painful. Alzheimer's disease patients may not recall everyone they have lost,

Jim sat morosely in his wheelchair. His speech came in fragments and was interrupted by long pauses, but the message was clear enough. ". . . some nice young folks. . . ." (He meant the student nurses who rotated through the unit each spring term.) "One came over . . . came a lot." He paused. "Asked her where it was—had to get it all ready—going to paint my room." Jim's hand trembled. "She said she'd help me. But they left . . . never came back." Later Jim said, "I can't get it ready by myself." Jim was experiencing the pain of trying to develop lasting relationships in a nursing home.

Illustration 2.4 Loss of Friends and Caregivers

A group of nursing home residents with middle-stage Alzheimer's disease often huddled in their wheelchairs in a small circle. Two topics seldom failed to bring forth some response: their mother's names, and memories of the first night they spent in the nursing home. "I heard a baby cry," said one frail lady. (She must have heard another resident crying from a nearby room.) "Had to sleep alone," added another. (The emotion was still keen.)

Illustration 2.5 Loss of Familiar Environments

but they sense the losses nonetheless. They grieve for loved ones, including their former selves, whom they cannot remember.

Grieving makes it difficult for elderly residents to invest in new communication partners. Starting over requires more energy than most elderly persons can muster. Furthermore, staff turnover, shift changes, and the frequent relocation of the residents make losses a daily, even hourly, occurrence. An Alzheimer's disease patient with any awareness senses this constant change or "loss" as troubling and confusing (Illustration 2.4).

6. *Loss of familiar environments.* For a nursing home resident, the ultimate symbol of helplessness and loss is losing one's own living quarters. New residents are assailed by unidentifiable sights, sounds, smells, and textures. They are distressed by having roommates instead of spouses, call bells instead of telephones, and trays instead of dishes. Uniforms, mimeographed menus, and fluorescent lighting constantly remind them that they are no longer at home. And every few hours, a new set of faces arrives. This explains why many Alzheimer's disease patients never reorient to their new surroundings (Illustration 2.5).

7. *Loss of first-language partners.* Many elderly nursing home residents do not share a first language with their fellow residents or with the direct care staff members. They may be immigrants for whom English is a second language, or they may be American-born but the staff is composed largely of individuals who speak English as a second language. Regardless of the situation, persons who are old and unwell find it increasingly difficult to speak or understand in their second language. They may resort to talking in their first language. They also have more trouble understanding any language that is spoken with a heavy accent. Caregivers who do not share the same first language with a patient face an extra challenge communicating when that person has Alzheimer's disease.

Quick Tip Summary: Communication Breakdowns
Caused by the Aging Process
Aging brings with it a host of physical, psychosocial, and environmental changes and losses. The result is that nursing home residents experience a drastic depletion in topics, places, and people needed for communication.

1. Loss of physical and financial independence.
2. Loss of livelihood and social role.
3. Loss of physical attractiveness and grooming skills.
4. Loss of energy.
5. Loss of family and friends.
6. Loss of familiar environments.
7. Loss of first-language partners.

COMMUNICATION ABILITIES PRESERVED UNTIL LATER STAGES OF ALZHEIMER'S DISEASE

In spite of language losses suffered by patients with Alzheimer's disease, many skills that support communication are remarkably preserved and remain for a long time. When working with Alzheimer's disease patients, caregivers should keep in mind six abilities that are nearly always preserved:

1. *The use of procedural memories.* Persons with Alzheimer's disease begin to lose memory for words, information, and events quite rapidly. But procedural memory, or the knowledge of how to perform familiar tasks, remains relatively intact until the later stages of dementia. Some scientists think this is because procedural memory is the most elemental of human

memory systems and is the only memory system capable of operating independently. This system sustains some very complex human activity—from walking and washing our hands to playing the piano and driving a car. Anderson[3] has explained that procedural memory is like a computer's program, whereas other types of memory are like the data stored in the computer. Alzheimer's disease patients begin to lose data rapidly, but the program still functions. They forget where they are going, but they still know how to walk; they forget what they are saying, but they still know how to talk. During the early stages of Alzheimer's disease, some patients are even able to learn new procedural memories. More specific examples of procedural memories include social rituals, such as passing plates, pouring coffee, or setting the table, and recreational activities, such as playing the piano or dancing. Although Alzheimer's disease patients can no longer plan a complete meal or master the subtlety of chess, they may still be able to mix batter and flip pancakes and to make the basic moves in checkers.

2. *The ability to access early life memories.* One phenomenon repeatedly mentioned by family caregivers is the ability of Alzheimer's disease patients to recall childhood memories better than information from more recent decades. Families are dismayed to note that while Dad cannot remember the names of his spouse of 45 years or any of his children, he easily recalls the name of his mother, who died when he was 12 years old. When asked to talk about his home, he describes not the house he built himself and in which he raised a family, but the house in which he was raised.

Earliest memories appear to be so "hard-wired" that they resist deterioration for a very long time. Some families find this upsetting and engage in endless efforts to bring their loved one back to the present: "No, Dad, your mother died when you were 12! Don't you remember Addie? Your wife, Addie? Our mother?" If they could accept and enjoy the old memories that their father can summon, they would find greater satisfaction in their conversations.

3. *The ability to recite, read aloud, and sing with good pronunciation and grammar.* Speech-language pathologists and linguists who have studied the language of Alzheimer's disease patients have observed that while these patients have little to say, they say it with good grammar. They can still respond automatically to greetings, recite prayers, and sing old songs. In fact, this automatic singing and speaking ability often brings them comfort and joy.

4. *The ability to engage in social ritual.* Alzheimer's disease patients retain the ability to use social ritual: "Please pass the sugar." "How are you today?" "Fine, thank you." "Would you like some coffee?" "No, thanks." In several studies that looked at the dining abilities of patients with Alzheimer's disease, subjects carried out social rituals—offering one another candy, making small talk—surprisingly well. Alzheimer's disease patients can exchange greetings, ask the time, excuse themselves, and accept compliments. The skill of taking turns during conversation is also maintained well into the middle stages of the disease.

5. *The desire for interpersonal communication.* Sometimes residents with Alzheimer's disease drive the staff crazy with their constant complaining and asking for things that they do not need. Their real need is for human contact. They may have learned that if they do not complain or demand, nobody talks to them. Most patients with Alzheimer's disease retain a strong desire to communicate until the late stages of the disease. In fact, a conversation study found that loss of the desire to communicate was a signal that the patient was passing into a more severe stage of the disease.[4]

6. *The desire for interpersonal respect.* The best evidence that Alzheimer's disease patients retain their desire for respect is how quickly they show resentment when treated with disdain by their caregivers. From the patients' point of view, lack of respect includes having caregivers talk to them or yell at them as if they were children, being ignored, being called by "pet" names without giving permission, being moved from place to place, or receiving medical treatment without explanation. Although their behavior may indeed be childlike and exasperating, Alzheimer's disease patients continue to expect to be treated as adults, and, in fact, react more positively and perform better when addressed as adults.

Quick Tip Summary: Communication Abilities Preserved in Patients through the Middle Stage of Alzheimer's Disease

1. The use of procedural memories.
2. The ability to access early life memories.
3. The ability to recite, read aloud, and sing with good pronunciation and grammar.
4. The ability to engage in social ritual.
5. The desire for interpersonal communication.
6. The desire for interpersonal respect.

SUCCESSFUL COMMUNICATION WITH ALZHEIMER'S DISEASE PATIENTS

REFERENCES

1. Van Riper C, Emerick L. Speech Correction: An Introduction to Speech Pathology and Audiology. Englewood Cliffs, NJ: Prentice-Hall, 1990;34.
2. Foy S, Mitchell M. Factors contributing to learned helplessness in the institutionalized aged: a literature review. Phys Occup Ther Geriatrics 1990;9(2):1.
3. Anderson, JR. Language, Memory, and Thought. Hillsdale, NJ: Lawrence Erlbaum Associates, 1990:
4. Santo Pietro MJ, DeCotiis E, McCarthy JM, Ostuni E. Conversations in Alzheimer's disease: implications of semantic and pragmatic breakdowns. Paper presented to the annual convention of the American Speech-Language-Hearing Association. Seattle, WA, 1990.

GOOD PRACTICE 2.1 COMMUNICATION ABILITIES LOST IN EARLY, MIDDLE, AND LATE STAGES OF ALZHEIMER'S DISEASE

Directions: The emergence of each of the communication symptoms below may indicate that the patient has entered a particular stage of the disease. Refer to Table 2.1 to determine which stage of the disease each symptom indicates. Check under the correct column.

Symptom	Early	Middle	Late
1. Patient first appears confused about the time of day.			
2. Patient makes mistakes that he or she no longer corrects.			
3. Patient no longer starts conversation.			
4. Patient speaks in jargon or is mute.			
5. Patient can read mechanically, but does not understand what is read.			
6. Patient no longer recognizes close family members.			
7. Patient has difficulty seeing things from another's point of view.			
8. Patient has little control over anger and argumentativeness.			
9. Patient cannot retain recent information.			
10. Patient cannot form any new memories.			

GOOD PRACTICE 2.2   CHARACTERISTIC CHANGES IN THE COMMUNICATION OF ALZHEIMER'S DISEASE PATIENTS

Directions: Identify the underlined words in residents' quotes below as examples of *empty speech, paraphasias, stereotypic phrases,* or *violations of conversational rules.* (Hint: some quotes might fit more than one category.)

	Empty speech	Para- phasia	Stereotypic phrase	Violation of conver- sational rules
1. "Oh no you don't. <u>I never was one for that kind of thing. No, I never went in for that kind of thing</u>."				
2. "I used to like to do <u>that</u>. We used to, you know, do <u>stuff like that</u> all the time."				
3. "I'm dying of the <u>cold</u> in here! Open the window; give us some cool air!"				
4. "Oh yes, I was always a big <u>foot-ball</u> fan. When I was little, my Dad took me to see Babe Ruth and the, you know, the Yankees."				
5. "<u>A mile a minute. A mile a minute</u>. Everybody nowadays goes a mile a minute."				

GOOD PRACTICE 2.3 ROLE PLAY OF COMMUNICATION BREAKDOWNS CAUSED BY THE AGING PROCESS

Directions: For each scenario, select a person to play the part of the resident and someone to play the part of the staff member. Explain to each individual what type of character he or she is to act out and the circumstances of the situation. If possible, set up the activity so that each role player knows how his or her character will act but not what the other person is going to do. After each scenario, discuss these two questions:

1. How did you feel in this situation?
2. How would you have preferred the other person to behave or respond?

Resident's role	Staff member's role
Scene 1	
Sadie is small, helpless, and whiny. She only talks about her ailments. She is confined to a wheelchair. She (thinks she) needs help with everything.	Susan has a strong personality and a large number of residents under her care. She is very efficient and wants to get Sadie to breakfast by 7:30 AM. It is now 7:25 AM.
Scene 2	
George is able to walk using his walker, but only slowly and with great care. He is very unsteady and needs to concentrate on each step.	Alana takes every opportunity to practice her English and she has a naturally friendly manner. She feels compelled to engage George in conversation on his long walk to the activity room.
Scene 3	
Hiram is feeling lonely and depressed. His familiar roommate has moved to another floor, he does not recognize his new aide, and his family has not come to visit in a long time. He doesn't want to do anything.	Barbara, the new aide, is kind and gentle. She has been told that Hiram needs to get out of his room more.

UNIT 3

Other Communication Disorders in Alzheimer's Disease Patients

---

UNIT OUTLINE

Premise

1. At least 50% of nursing home residents have significant communication disorders unrelated to dementia.
2. Patients with Alzheimer's disease suffer from these disorders at a higher rate than other elderly persons.
3. This unit will help caregivers understand these additional stresses on a patient's communication system and explain how to compensate for them whenever possible.

Definitions

    Speech

    Language

    Voice

    Hearing

**How to Recognize and Compensate for Other
         Communication Disorders**

    Sensory Impairments

      1. Hearing impairment, recruitment, and ringing in the ears (tinnitus)
      2. Vision disorders and blindness

    Speech and Language Disabilities

      1. Aphasia
      2. Dysarthria and dysphagia
      3. Voice problems
      4. Tracheostomy

    Medical Problems

      1. Chronic illness
      2. Drug and medication problems
      3. Problems with oral hygiene and nutrition

PREMISE

According to estimates, at least 50% of all nursing home residents have significant communication disorders that are unrelated to dementia, and Alzheimer's disease patients suffer from these disorders at a higher rate than other elderly persons.[1] In addition, many nursing home residents have medical disabilities that weaken their communication skills. The presence of Alzheimer's disease makes treatment of these other disorders more, rather than less, imperative. Additional handicaps should not be dismissed with the attitude, "Well, she has dementia. No sense worrying about that hearing problem." If a patient is doubly communication handicapped, then he or she is doubly hard to reach. This unit is designed to aid caregivers in understanding and reducing the impact of these additional stresses on a patient's communication system.

DEFINITIONS

Before describing these additional disorders, this unit will review the components of the communication process discussed in Units 1 and 2.

Speech

Speech is how the words sound when a person talks. Are they clearly spoken? Slurred? Misarticulated? Does the person say "sue" for "shoe" or "nursh" for "nurse"? Ordinarily, if Alzheimer's disease patients do not have additional communication disorders, their speech does not deteriorate until the final stages of the disease.

Language

Language is composed of vocabulary, grammar, and intention to communicate. Sentences are put together with words and grammar to express ideas and feelings. Language breakdown in Alzheimer's disease patients begins early and worsens as they become more cognitively impaired.

Voice

Voice is the sound produced by the vibrations of the vocal cords within the larynx, or "voice box," in the throat. The sound of the voice indicates whether the speaker is a man, a woman, an older person, or a child. Voice reveals the health, emotion, and purpose of the speaker.

Hearing

Hearing is a sensory process. Hearing depends on the proper functioning of all three parts of the ear: the outer ear and ear canal, which gather sound; the middle ear, which contains three tiny bones that transfer sound from the outer ear to the auditory nerve; and the inner ear, the nerve center that converts sound to impulses that the brain interprets and to which it responds. Adequate hearing is essential to understanding the communication of others. Adequate hearing is also important in the production of good, clear speech. Persons who cannot hear their own speech gradually lose precise articulation and may speak with a voice that is too soft or too loud.

HOW TO RECOGNIZE AND COMPENSATE FOR OTHER COMMUNICATION DISORDERS

Communication disorders experienced by aging persons with Alzheimer's disease are divided into three subsets: (1) sensory impairments, (2) speech and language disabilities, and (3) medical problems. Coping with the additional communication problems of patients with Alzheimer's disease is easier if the underlying causes are understood.

Sensory Impairments

1. *Hearing impairment, recruitment, and ringing in the ears (tinnitus).* Impaired hearing is a serious and common communication problem among persons with Alzheimer's disease. More than one-half of all Americans older than 65 years have significant hearing impairments; however, the incidence of hearing loss among patients with Alzheimer's disease may be as much as 20% higher than the incidence among normal elderly persons.[2, 3]

a. Clean wax and hair from ears. Check for water trapped in the ear canal after the patient has shampooed or showered.

b. Be alert to signs of fluid buildup in the middle ear (especially after an allergy attack or upper respiratory illness); redness of the ear canal; a painful reaction to touch around the ear; "quiet" speech; and instances of increased misunderstanding or nonresponse to the speech of others. These symptoms should be reported to the patient's physician.

c. Establish eye contact with the patient before speaking. Speak more slowly but do not exaggerate lip movements. Speak more loudly but lower the pitch of your voice. A lower pitched voice is more easily understood by persons with hearing loss.

RECOMMENDATION 3.1 Recommendations for Helping Alzheimer's Disease Patients Who Have Conductive Hearing Loss

Even an otherwise healthy individual who has a hearing loss may find the constant effort to understand others exhausting. Many people become suspicious and depressed and withdraw from social contact when suffering from an untreated hearing loss. When a resident with Alzheimer's disease has a significant hearing loss, communication with that person will be much more difficult.

Conductive hearing loss results from malfunctions of the outer ear or middle ear. It might occur from wax buildup in the ear canal, inflammation of the ear canal (swimmer's ear), a buildup of fluid behind the ear drum caused by allergies or upper respiratory infections, or a buildup of bony material in the ear (otosclerosis). A conductive hearing loss leads to "fuzzy" hearing or a feeling of pressure or pain in the ears (Recommendation 3.1).

Sensorineural hearing loss, or "nerve deafness," results from a malfunction of the inner ear or auditory nerve. It can be caused by long exposure to loud noise (e.g., machinery, gunfire, or loud music), a high fever, certain medications, or old age itself (presbycusis). People with sensorineural hearing losses have trouble distinguishing many of the consonant sounds that give speech its clarity. They hear the speaker talking but cannot understand the words. Sensorineural hearing losses can seldom be treated medically, but they can often be helped with hearing aids properly fitted by an audiologist.

Many elderly persons who have nerve deafness suffer from *recruitment*. A person with recruitment might not hear soft speech at all, but shouting causes the auditory system to suddenly "kick in," and the person hears the shout at its true level of loudness, causing him or her to jump and complain.

a. Do not try to talk to the person against a noisy background. Close the door, take the patient to a quieter area, or turn down the radio.

b. Establish eye contact with the patient before speaking. Speak more slowly. Lower your pitch, but use a normal, not a louder tone of voice. Never shout at a person who has sensorineural hearing loss.

c. If the patient has a hearing aid, encourage him or her to wear it. Learn to fit the earpiece snugly into the ear canal, to find the best settings, and to check for dead batteries.

d. Learn how to maintain the hearing aid: clean the tubing, replace batteries, and check for air leaks, which cause the aid to whistle or squeak.

RECOMMENDATION 3.2   Recommendations for Helping Alzheimer's Disease Patients Who Have Sensorineural Hearing Loss

A number of people with nerve deafness also suffer from incessant ringing in the ears or *tinnitus*. Tinnitus not only is extremely distracting to its victims, it also interferes with the ability to hear what others are saying. Persons with tinnitus are very uncomfortable in noisy settings (e.g., televisions playing, people talking, or trays clattering). The noise distracts and annoys them and increases the tinnitus (Recommendation 3.2).

2. *Vision disorders and blindness.* Loss of vision constitutes a significant barrier to good communication. Vision that is clouded by cataracts, glaucoma, macular degeneration, loss of acuity, and unused eyeglasses increases an Alzheimer's disease patient's uncertainty about a speaker's identity. Clouded vision can also interfere with the reading of a speaker's facial expressions, and important information about a speaking partner's appearance and body language is lost.

As their disease progresses, many Alzheimer's patients are able to read written words long after they have lost the ability to understand spoken language. But if they have untreated visual impairments, they will be unable to use written words as an aid to better functioning (Recommendation 3.3).

Speech and Language Disabilities

1. *Aphasia.* Aphasia is a language problem that generally results from a stroke or other injury to the left side of the brain. Aphasic patients have difficulty in understanding and expressing language. Some patients have difficulty in the auditory compre-

> **a.** Be alert to the possibility that visual problems might account for a resident's apparent disorientation to place and time. Be sure that each patient's vision has been checked.
>
> **b.** Be sure that printed material and signs are in large, bold print and well-lighted. (See also Unit 4.)
>
> **c.** Check that eyeglasses are well-fitted, clean, and worn by the patient.

RECOMMENDATION 3.3 Recommendations for Helping Alzheimer's Disease Patients Overcome Visual Problems

hension of language but are able to speak fluently (*fluent* or *Wernicke's aphasia*). Others struggle to say one word at a time but appear to understand language fairly well (*nonfluent* or *Broca's aphasia*). The most common type of aphasia affecting elderly persons is *global aphasia*, or the severe loss of the ability to receive and express language.[4]

Persons with aphasia often have weakness or paralysis on the right side of the body (*hemiplegia*), and a loss of vision in the right visual field of each eye (*hemianopsia*). Many stroke survivors are *labile*, crying or laughing at the slightest provocation. Persons with aphasia can be expected to react with anger out of frustration because they can no longer speak with ease.

When a person suffers a series of small strokes, or *transient ischemic attacks* (TIAs), the result may be not only a mild aphasia, but also a *multi-infarct dementia* (MID). MID closely resembles Alzheimer's disease in everything but its progression. Alzheimer's disease follows a steady downhill course, whereas the person with MID tends to plateau until the next series of small strokes.

The language problems of aphasia are different from those of Alzheimer's disease. Aphasia does not typically create problems with reasoning and remembering or cause disorientation or personality changes as does Alzheimer's disease. An aphasic patient is often acutely aware of his or her limitations; the Alzheimer's disease patient who has moved beyond the early stages of disease is not so aware. Most aphasic patients, no matter how old or how long post-onset, respond well to direct, patient-centered communication intervention by a speech-language pathologist. The most effective communication interventions with Alzheimer's disease patients, however, must focus on improving the communication styles of caregivers and providing environmental supports and activities to help maintain declining language skills as long as possible (Recommendation 3.4).

> **a.** Position yourself in the patient's visual field, usually on the patient's left side.
>
> **b.** Get the person's attention before speaking, e.g., sit at eye level, hold the person's hands, or say the person's name.
>
> **c.** Speak slowly and clearly and use short sentences. Allow the tone of your voice and manner of touch to convey emotional support.
>
> **d.** Give the patient time to respond. Respect any attempts to verbalize; strongly reinforce the patient's nonverbal responses, such as hand squeezing, pointing, or directed gaze.
>
> **e.** Talk to the patient and provide plenty of opportunities for the patient to observe, if not to engage in, communication with others.

RECOMMENDATION 3.4 Recommendations for Communicating with an Alzheimer's Disease Patient Who Is Also Aphasic

2. *Dysarthria and dysphagia.* A speech problem caused by muscle weakness resulting from nerve damage is called *dysarthria*. Nerve damage may result from stroke, tumors, trauma, viruses, toxic poisoning, or degenerative conditions, such as Parkinson's disease. Symptoms of dysarthria vary widely depending on which part of the nervous system is damaged. Some patients develop slurred speech and a nasal voice quality, whereas others strain to produce any speech at all. Speech might sound uneven, sporadic, even drunk, or it might be breathy, rapid, monotonous, and barely audible.

Patients with muscle weaknesses of the face, the mouth, or the throat may also have trouble controlling saliva, chewing, or swallowing (*dysphagia*). Symptoms of dysphagia may include some or all of the following: (a) choking on food or drink; (b) a wet, gurgly voice; (c) an extended period of chewing followed by difficulty triggering a swallow; (d) chronic drooling or facial droop; and (e) low-grade fever signaling aspiration pneumonia. As with aphasia, dysarthria and dysphagia can be treated successfully by speech-language pathologists who teach muscle strengthening exercises and compensatory ways to communicate and swallow effectively (Recommendation 3.5).

3. *Voice problems.* The most underreported communication disorders in the nursing home are voice problems.[5] General frailty, neurologic deterioration, injury, or weakness can make an older person's voice so soft it cannot be heard. Years of smoking, drinking, or using medical or recreational drugs; chronic upper respiratory disease; or prolonged screaming or crying can leave a patient's voice hoarse and difficult to understand. The voices of elderly persons can also be monotonous, shaky, or intermittent.

a. Give the patient plenty of time to speak.

b. Speak slowly and encourage the patient to do likewise. Many dysarthric persons sound clearer if they can control their rate of speaking.

c. Provide the dysarthric patient with firm hip, trunk, and head support for speech as well as for eating. Patients speak best when they are sitting in an upright, firmly supported position.

d. Monitor closely dysarthric patients for signs of difficulty with swallowing. Any changes should be reported immediately to the patient's physician.

e. Follow all feeding instructions carefully and record observed swallowing problems.

RECOMMENDATION 3.5   Recommendations for Helping Alzheimer's Disease Patients Who Have Dysarthria or Dysphagia

a. Provide good upright trunk and head support during those times when the resident is preparing to speak. Patients who are slumped sideways in their chairs or beds have a harder time getting enough breath and muscle support for strong voicing.

b. Eliminate background noise and interruptions in places and at times when conversation among residents is likely to occur. Do not force them to compete with noise, such as a television or clattering dishes.

c. Use simple, positive reinforcement and reminders for speaking louder and more clearly: "Ah Mabel, you are in good voice today!" "Charlie, please speak up. Sara wants to hear about your daughter's visit."

d. Listen to patients' voices after mealtimes to make sure their throats are free of bits of food that make the voice sound "wet," and instruct the patient to swallow or to clear the throat.

RECOMMENDATION 3.6   Recommendations for Supporting Alzheimer's Disease Patients Who Have Voice Problems

Since a large percentage of elderly persons do not hear well, those who cannot speak loudly enough to be heard by the other residents are at an enormous disadvantage during conversation. Of greater importance, if a patient calls for help and cannot be heard, that resident's very life might be at risk. Some voice problems can be treated successfully by a physician or a speech-language pathologist. Others might benefit from a portable microphone and amplifier (Recommendation 3.6).

a. Eliminate background noise so that the patient can be more easily heard.

b. Use simple verbal reminders and perhaps physical cues to help the patient remember to cover the stoma before speaking: "George, use your finger. Cover your stoma."

c. Use your own gloved finger to cover the stoma if the patient is unable to do so. Allow the patient to inhale and then apply gentle pressure while he or she speaks a few words on exhalation.

d. Keep a "magic slate" or pad and pen available at bedside.

RECOMMENDATION 3.7 Recommendations for Making Communication Easier for a Tracheotomized Resident with Alzheimer's Disease

4. *Tracheostomy.* Patients who breathe through tracheostomy tubes have a special type of speech-voice disorder. The air they breathe is not exhaled through the vocal cords and out of the mouth. They cannot produce voice unless the opening, or stoma, is completely covered by a finger or two or unless they have had a valve (e.g., Passy-Muir) implanted. A resident with a "trach" needs special medical care and special help with communication. First, these patients have great difficulty producing audible voices under the best of circumstances. Second, they may need help to activate what little voice they do have. Many elderly patients do not have the dexterity to adequately cover the stomas themselves. Most Alzheimer's disease patients must be reminded to do so (Recommendation 3.7).

Medical Problems

1. *Chronic illness.* New admissions to nursing homes have an average of four co-occurring illnesses. Most frequently these are diabetes, arthritis, heart disease, atherosclerosis, osteoporosis, emphysema, cancer, or Parkinson's disease. Alzheimer's disease patients also suffer from these medical conditions. Beyond the stresses of dementia, such illnesses drain their energy and receptiveness, making good communication with professional caregivers even more difficult. Knowing the effects of an individual's medical problems can help you estimate the extent to which illness interferes with communication (Recommendation 3.8).

2. *Drug and medication problems.* One of the most common impairments in communication among the elderly is caused by medication. When assessing a resident's communication impairment, the direct effects and the side effects of medications must be taken into

> **a.** Gear your expectations of a patient's communication ability to the patient's level of illness.
>
> **b.** Schedule important moments of communication when the patient is most alert and comfortable.

RECOMMENDATION 3.8 Recommendations for Communicating with Alzheimer's Disease Patients with Chronic Illnesses

	If the patient is taking:	Look for:
a.	Antihistamines, antiseizure medications, antidepressants	Painfully dry mouth, sore and bleeding gums, agitation
b.	Steroids	Slurred speech
c.	Cardiac medications	Drowsiness
d.	Aspirin, chemotherapies	Ringing in the ears (tinnitus), hearing loss
e.	Psychotropic drugs	Nervous tics, involuntary movements, difficulty opening the jaw to eat or speak
f.	Sleeping pills, tranquilizers, pain killers	Disorientation, memory loss, slurred speech, drowsiness

RECOMMENDATION 3.9 Recommendations for Recognizing the Effects of Medication on Communication[6]

account. Elderly patients with chronic conditions are highly vulnerable to the long-term effects of drugs, and furthermore, because they suffer from multiple medical conditions, they are often victims of toxic drug interactions. They are also more likely than younger persons to have atypical reactions to drugs. Sometimes the effects of medications masquerade as primary illnesses—depression, anemia, confusion, and dementia (Recommendation 3.9).

3. *Problems with oral hygiene and nutrition.* Tooth decay, poorly fitting or absent dentures, dry mouth (*xerostomia*), or sores in the mouth affect how much a person feels like talking and how well he or she talks. Someone fighting the problems of loose dentures and sore gums may not want to eat or talk. A vicious circle begins: not eating causes major weight loss, which in turn causes dentures to shift and fit less well. This condition creates even more discomfort and further lessens the desire for eating and communication. Nutrition problems are also caused by persistent swallowing problems (*dysphagia*), illness, or a poor diet. Whatever the cause, when

> **a.** Insist on good oral hygiene and advocate regular dental consults.
>
> **b.** Know where the patient's dentures are kept. Make sure they are cleaned and placed in the patient's mouth correctly and comfortably.
>
> **c.** Report suspected nutrition problems immediately.

RECOMMENDATION 3.10 Recommendations for Preventing Communication Problems Caused by Poor Oral Hygiene and Nutrition

nutrition is significantly compromised, then speech, energy, and health are severely at risk.

A resident's pain from cavities, food lodged in the gums, cold sores, or ill-fitting dentures should never be underestimated. Anyone who has had even the tiniest canker sore on the tip of the tongue knows how painful and how distracting it can be. Patients with poorly tended gums and teeth are at greater risk for bacterial infections, which create changes in blood coagulation variables. These changes could help trigger a stroke.[7] Finally, social communication opportunities are lost because of the chronic bad breath caused by inadequate mouth care. Other people are not as likely to come close to or linger with residents who have halitosis (Recommendation 3.10).

4. *Clinical depression.* The primary symptoms of depression are withdrawal and impaired communication. Research indicates that those who have least control over their own lives (e.g., nursing home residents) experience the most stress and depression. Most residents suffer from depression at some time during their nursing home stay,[8] and nearly all persons with early- to middle-stage Alzheimer's disease experience depression. Yet, elderly persons in nursing homes have little contact with mental health specialists. Even though a resident is old or suffers from Alzheimer's disease, direct treatment or counseling for depression and stress should be made available. Direct treatment could relieve the symptoms of a communication disorder resulting from depression (Recommendation 3.11).

5. *Balance and movement problems.* Staying balanced and moving about safely are very real challenges for many nursing home residents. Arthritis, osteoporosis, paralysis, pain, weakness, and fear of falling all contribute to communication problems. For example, limitations in movement and balance decrease the ability of residents to groom themselves. Washing, styling hair, shaving, or putting on makeup all take an agility that patients with Alzheimer's disease no longer have. Balance and movement problems also play a major role in restricting the patient's communication opportunities in other ways. Patients who have a limited ability to move may have

---

a. Advocate mental health consults for patients who appear chronically or severely depressed.

b. Do not assume someone can be "jollied" out of depression.

c. Without demanding it, encourage residents to participate in activities and discourage isolation.

RECOMMENDATION 3.11   Recommendations for Reducing the Effects of Depression on the Communication of Alzheimer's Disease Patients

---

a. Consider canes, wheelchairs, and willing escorts as communication aids as well as physical supports, and encourage their use.

b. Begin transport to social events early to allow on-time arrival and comfortable seating.

RECOMMENDATION 3.12   Recommendations for Reducing the Effects of Balance and Movement Problems on Communication of Alzheimer's Disease Patients

difficulty turning to face a speaker and therefore may miss the message. A person with poor balance must pay more attention to avoiding a fall than to listening to someone speak. An Alzheimer's disease patient who cannot get around because of balance and movement problems is at higher risk for isolation, withdrawal, depression, and more rapid deterioration (Recommendation 3.12).

Quick Tip Summary: Communication Breakdowns Resulting from Sensory Impairments, Speech and Language Disabilities, or Medical Problems Not Related to Alzheimer's Disease
Elderly nursing home residents have a variety of problems that negatively affect their desire and ability to communicate. If residents have Alzheimer's disease as well, their problems are more than doubled.

A. Sensory Impairments
1. More than one-half of persons older than 65 years have a significant *hearing loss.* Conductive hearing loss can often be treated medically; sensorineural hearing loss can frequently be helped with hearing aids. Some hearing-impaired patients also suffer from recruitment (sensitivity to loud noises) and tinnitus (ringing in the ears).
2. *Vision disorders* constitute a significant barrier to communication. Cataracts, glaucoma, macular degeneration, loss of acu-

ity, and unused eyeglasses interfere with the ability of Alzheimer's disease patients to understand speakers because facial expression and body language cannot be discerned. Alzheimer's disease patients with untreated visual impairments are also unable to benefit from their retained ability to read written words.

B. *Speech and Language Disabilities*
  1. *Aphasia* is a breakdown in the understanding and expression of language caused by damage to the left side of the brain. Aphasia affects language differently from Alzheimer's disease.
  2. *Dysarthria* is a weakness in the speech muscles that results from neurologic damage caused by stroke, illness, or injury. Symptoms include hypernasality, unnaturally slow or rapid speech, and imprecise pronunciation. Some dysarthric patients also exhibit dysphagia (swallowing problems).
  3. *Voice disorders* afflict many nursing home residents. Their voices are often too weak or too hoarse to be easily heard, especially by other residents who have hearing losses. Poor postural support aggravates a weak voice.
  4. *Tracheostomy* patients must cover their stomas to speak or must have special valves inserted to allow vocalization.

C. *Medical Problems*
  1. The *chronic illnesses* of nursing home residents—diabetes, arthritis, heart disease, atherosclerosis, emphysema, etc.—interfere greatly with the patient's energy level for communication.
  2. *Drug and medication problems* may present as primary communication problems. Watch for symptoms, such as slurring, dry painful mouth, or confusion, which might be connected to causes, such as medication side effects, overdoses, or interactions.
  3. *Problems with oral hygiene and nutrition* can lead to painful mouth, halitosis, or weakness, all of which interfere with communication.
  4. *Clinical depression* occurs in many nursing home residents and in most patients in the early and middle stages of Alzheimer's disease.
  5. *Balance and movement problems* make it difficult for residents to participate in activities and to attend to speakers.

COPING WITH SUDDEN CHANGES IN COMMUNICATION PATTERNS

Sudden changes in a resident's communication pattern can be an important signal to staff members that something is wrong. The

Table 3.1   How to Respond to Sudden Changes in Speech

Communication changes	Possible communication solutions
Speech becomes slurred; words are indistinct, "mumbly."	Could be sign of impending stroke or reaction to medication. OR, patient may not be using hearing aid or dentures. **Investigate and report as a precaution.**
Patient might be unable to speak; might show facial droop or drooling.	**Report to charge nurse or physician immediately.**

ability to interpret a sudden change could avert a medical or emotional crisis.

Sudden Changes in Speech

If a patient's speech is suddenly harder to hear or understand, or if words are mumbled or missing, or if speech is stuttered or lacking altogether, the patient may be entering a later stage of Alzheimer's disease. However, these symptoms might also signal one of the problems listed in Table 3.1.

Sudden Changes in Language

If a resident is suddenly "rude" when he or she had previously joined in social communication, if a resident rapidly changes from talking occasionally to becoming almost mute, or if language that was once functional suddenly becomes full of hallucinations, then the cause of the change should be investigated (Table 3.2).

Sudden Changes in Voice

If a patient exhibits unexpected changes in voice quality, some process independent of Alzheimer's disease is operating. The change should be taken seriously and addressed (Table 3.3).

Table 3.2   How to Respond to Sudden Changes in Language

Communication changes	Possible communication solutions
Conversational rudeness increases; attempts to communicate in previously functional ways decrease.	May need more social conversational opportunities to stimulate and maintain current communication ability.
Communication and/or behavior patterns go from reasonably compliant to agitated, repetitive, even combative.	May signal pain or impending illness; need different level of activity; OR, may benefit from more staff attention and social communication.
Reverts to first language.	Not unusual for elderly patients. Ask family to teach staff a few words in the patient's first language; write important words on index cards, e.g., "bathroom" and "hungry." Bring in taped music sung in the native tongue to calm and entertain the patient; locate staff member or volunteer who speaks the same language.
Becomes restless or distraught during group activities that were formerly enjoyed.	Language level of group may now be too complex. Simplify language; slow down rate of speech. Decrease longer conversations; increase the number of short (e.g., 30-second) exchanges.
Becomes mute or near mute with no other signs of deterioration due to disease. Appears more withdrawn; eats less.	May be depressed. Try more one-on-one communication and acceptance of complaints or distress. Seek counseling for patient. OR, may have sores in mouth caused by ill-fitting dentures or by excessively dry mouth. **Report to charge nurse or physician immediately.** Resident is at risk for bacterial infection.
Increases cursing, swearing, or use of abusive language.	May be a sign of mental decline or emotional upset. Do not take abuse personally. Look for physical, emotional, or environmental causes. Listen for the real emotional message behind the tirade.
Language suddenly becomes "wild" or hallucinatory.	**Report to charge nurse or physician immediately.** Look for drug reactions or interactions. Seek to eliminate auditory or visual overload.

Table 3.3 How to Respond to Sudden Changes in Voice

Communication changes	Possible communication solutions
Voice becomes very weak or "wobbly"; more difficult to hear.	**Monitor carefully.** May be a sign of physical deterioration or illness.
Voice is wet-sounding or "gurgly," especially after eating or drinking.	**Report immediately.** May signal swallowing problems. Must be monitored closely to guard against aspiration.
Voice remains hoarse or "raspy" for 3 weeks or longer.	**Report immediately.** A chronically hoarse voice may signal a serious condition, such as polyps or cancer of the vocal cords.

REFERENCES

1. Fein DJ. The prevalence of speech and language impairments. ASHA 1983;25(2):37.
2. Weinstein B, Amsel L. Hearing loss and senile dementia in the institutionalized elderly. Clin Gerontol 1986;4:3.
3. Gilhome-Herbst KG, Humphrey C. Hearing impairment and mental state in the elderly living at home. BMJ 1980;281:903.
4. Tonkovich JD. Communication Disorders in the Elderly. In B Shadden (ed), Communication Behavior and Aging: A Source Book for Clinicians. Baltimore: Williams & Wilkins, 1988;200.
5. Colton RH, Casper JK. Understanding Voice Problems: A Physiological Perspective for Diagnosis and Treatment. Baltimore: Williams & Wilkins, 1996;5.
6. Vogel D, Carter JE. Effects of Drugs on Communication Disorders. San Diego: Singular, 1994.
7. Valtonen V. Infection as a risk factor for infarction and atherosclerosis. Ann Med 1991;23:539.
8. Folstein MF, McHugh PR. Dementia Syndrome of Depression. In R Katzman, RD Terry, K Bick (eds), Alzheimer's Disease: Senile Dementia and Related Disorders. New York: Raven, 1978;87.

GOOD PRACTICE 3.1   RESPONDING TO OTHER COMMUNICATION PROBLEMS OR SUDDEN CHANGES IN COMMUNICATION ABILITIES

Directions: Based on information in Unit 3, complete these scenarios:

1. One morning, Alf's speech was very slurred and "mumbly." He was also drooling slightly from the right side of his mouth. You should_____
because_____.

2. Rhoda is a Holocaust survivor who came to the United States after World War II. Today, most of her words are in Polish or Yiddish. To make her happier and your job easier, you could _____
_____.

3. Vera is bedridden, has no speech and must have her pureed diet spoon-fed to her each meal. During feeding sessions, she often moans and makes primitive noises that have a wet, "gargly" sound. She sounds congested and coughs frequently. You should_____
_____ because_____.

4. Asher's conversations with you have become increasingly "wild" and hallucinatory. Some of the things he says are scary. You should_____.

5. Angelina has a very hoarse, "raspy" voice. She has been in your charge for 15 months and has always sounded this way. You should_____.

GOOD PRACTICE 3.2   CASE STUDY OF A COMMUNICATION-IMPAIRED RESIDENT

Directions: Identify a resident in your facility with whom you have difficulty communicating. Fill in the background information to the best of your knowledge. Provide a brief description of each of the communication problems listed in the guidelines below.

Initials of Resident:_____ Age:_____ Sex:_____

First Language:_____ Level of Education:_____

Previous Occupation:_____

General Background Information: (date of admission, family history, etc.)_____

_____

_____

I. Communication Problems Caused by Sensory Impairments:
   Hearing impairment or tinnitus_____
   Vision disorders_____
II. Communication Problems Caused by Speech and Language
      Disabilities:
   Aphasia_____
   Dysarthria or dysphagia_____
   Voice disorders_____
   Tracheostomy_____
III. Communication Breakdowns Caused by Medical Problems:
   Chronic illnesses_____
   Drugs and medication problems_____
   Problems with oral hygiene and nutrition_____
   Clinical depression_____
   Balance and movement problems_____
IV. Communication Problems Caused by the Aging Process:
   Loss of independence_____
   Loss of livelihood and social role_____
   Loss of physical attractiveness_____
   Loss of energy_____
   Loss of family and friends_____
   Loss of familiar environments_____
   Loss of first-language partners_____
V. Communication Breakdowns Caused by Alzheimer's Disease:
   Problems with memory_____
   Problems with understanding_____

Problems with expressive language_____

Problems with social skills_____

Empty speech; stereotypical/repetitive speech?_____

Mutism? Continual crying out?_____

VI. Reducing Communication Problems for the Resident:
How could you reduce the resident's communication
problems due to

Sensory impairments?_____

_____

Speech and language disabilities?_____

_____

Medical problems?_____

_____

Aging process?_____

_____

Alzheimer's disease?_____

_____

UNIT 4

Effects of the Physical Environment on Communication and Recommendations for Improving Environmental Factors

UNIT OUTLINE

Premise

1. Environmental factors can magnify the communication problems of patients with Alzheimer's disease.
2. Adjustments to the environment can have a positive effect on a patient's willingness and ability to communicate.

Definitions

Communication-impaired environment

Physical environment

Creating a Nursing Home Environment
    Conducive to Communication

Factors Interfering with Good Vision

1. Poorly arranged or inadequate lighting
2. Lack of visual accessibility
3. Missing or inadequate signage and information displays
4. Too little visual stimulation
5. Too much visual stimulation or clutter

Factors Interfering with Good Hearing

1. Too much ambient noise
2. Lack of proper amplification where sound and voice need to be heard
3. Lack of pleasurable or soothing auditory stimulation; lack of familiar sounds and voices

PREMISE

The less competent the individual, the greater the impact of environmental factors on that individual.[1]

[T]he biological, psychological, and social impairments of older people in our society make them selectively more vulnerable to environmental pressures than younger people.[2]

The environment affects individuals and individuals affect their surroundings. The environment is not simply a passive backdrop in which older people live, but an active contributor to what older persons will do and how well they will function.[3]

As these quotes emphasize, environmental factors can magnify the communication problems of patients with Alzheimer's disease. At the same time, communication problems of Alzheimer's disease patients can contribute to the unpleasantness of the environment. Adjustments to the environment can have a positive effect on a patient's willingness and ability to communicate. This unit examines the ways in which the physical environment of a nursing home have a negative impact on residents' faculties of vision, hearing, taste, and smell, and it will explore solutions to the resulting communication problems.

DEFINITIONS

Communication-Impaired Environment
"A communication-impaired environment is one where there are few opportunities for successful, meaningful communication."[3]

Physical Environment

The physical environment is made up of the nursing home buildings and grounds and all the objects that are contained within. Physical environment also refers to the way space is used and decorated, and to the sights, sounds, smells, tastes, and touches that each place uniquely communicates.

CREATING A NURSING HOME ENVIRONMENT CONDUCIVE TO COMMUNICATION

This unit offers examples of communication problems seen in many nursing homes that are a result of the physical environment. A number of recommendations are offered to offset or eliminate these problems. Not every recommendation will work in every setting or for every patient (for example, putting up poster-sized photographs of relatives has proved to be a reassuring visual reminder for some patients, but frightening for others). However, the list provides ideas for solutions that could reduce the number of communication problems in your facility.

Most of these solutions will work better if they are set into motion by the staff members who work directly and daily with Alzheimer's disease patients. Also, implementation of most of these solutions costs little or no money. Some, however, do take time. At first glance, an investment of time may seem to be a greater obstacle than an investment of money. Be patient! If you can implement even a few of these suggested changes, eventually your time and the institution's money will be saved. And the quality of your caregiving skills will increase immeasurably.

A final word of advice: It is not enough to change the environment to promote good communication and consider the job done. To prevent a gradual return of a communication-impaired environment, the direct care staff should have a procedure for regularly monitoring physical space and operational policies.

Factors Interfering with Good Vision

1. *Poorly arranged or inadequate lighting.* When lighting is inadequate or poorly arranged (for example, when there is glaring, unfiltered light or when shiny surfaces reflect light), patients must make a great effort to read facial cues, recognize words on signs, or enjoy pictures. They find it hard to gauge distances and depth. Inadequate or glaring light makes it difficult for them to find their way and reduces their enjoyment of activities. Patients who must concentrate on safety pay less attention to communication. By inter-

a. Lower table lamps and eliminate bare bulbs. Increase the number and location of lights. (Note: the recommended lighting level for elderly persons is 50–100 foot-candles.)[4]

b. Allow residents to operate lights in their personal spaces whenever possible. Choose lighting controls that are touch sensitive, easy to press, or operated by remote control. If feasible, place controls within the patient's reach.[4]

c. Avoid high-gloss finishes, even in visitors' areas. Minimize table glare with table coverings.

d. Remind staff members, family members, and volunteers to use good lighting when speaking to residents. Make sure that the light source is on the speaker's face and behind the listener. For example, raise window shades or drapes before group meetings, then seat the residents with their backs to the light.

e. Use floor and wall colors that absorb, rather than reflect light, e.g., beige walls and royal blue floors brighten and add contrast to the environment.

RECOMMENDATION 4.1   Recommendations for Improving Lighting

a. Position the head of the patient's bed so that the patient can see what is going on in the hallway. The patient will be more likely to see persons entering the room and be less startled when visitors approach the bed. If the patient needs to have the door closed to prevent wandering, install a dutch door and leave the top open.[3]

b. If the patient's room has a bathroom, place a "Bathroom" sign on its door. Leave the door open as a reminder to patients to use the toilet. Large "Bathroom" signs and open doors are helpful even for common/group bathrooms.

RECOMMENDATION 4.2   Recommendations for Improving Visual Accessibility

fering with sensory input, poor lighting increases patient fatigue and agitation (Recommendation 4.1).

2. *Lack of visual accessibility.* When patients cannot see the nurses' station or people passing their doors, they may become isolated, frightened, or paranoid. Patients who cannot see the bathroom are less likely to remember to use it; incontinence increases (Recommendation 4.2).

a. Place all identifying room labels and announcements at eye level.

b. Include personal photographs on nameplates at the entrance to patients' rooms and in areas where personal items are stored or displayed.

c. Color-code signs, name tags, symbols, and doorways. Knowing that the "Ladies Room" door is always pink and that the dietary workers are always dressed in blue can be extremely helpful to patients.

d. Avoid cluttered bulletin boards and wordy announcements. Make signs with black magic markers on off-white or pale pastel backgrounds. Print in large, bold, lower-case lettering. Limit messages to one, two, or three words.

e. Wear giant name tags with large, bold print. Point to your name when greeting a resident. Say your name and the Alzheimer's disease patient's name frequently.

f. Keep the resident's eye glasses clean.

RECOMMENDATION 4.3 Recommendations for Improving Signs and Information Displays

3. *Missing or inadequate signage and information displays.* Inadequate signage, missing signs, signs with small or illegible print, or signs with too much print promote wandering because patients cannot easily find their way. Small print on name tags, bulletin boards, and directories makes it impossible for patients to read and retain the names of caregivers, places, and events, and limits freedom of access to information, activities, and better "communication places" (Recommendation 4.3).

4. *Too little visual stimulation.* When there is too little visual stimulation, patients have fewer things to talk about. Their responsiveness to visual stimuli deteriorates more rapidly and they have fewer reminders of memories and family. Nutrition can also be affected by a lack of visual stimulation. Food that is presented in a boring way decreases appetite (Recommendation 4.4).

5. *Too much visual stimulation or clutter.* Visual overstimulation and clutter lead to agitation, stress, distraction, and confusion for staff members and residents (Recommendation 4.5).

Factors Interfering with Good Hearing

1. *Too much ambient noise.* Noise hinders successful communication. Too much noise can result from (a) the nature of building materials (e.g., lack of sound-absorbing materials); (b) the arrange-

---

a. Allow plenty of visual and physical access to the out-of-doors.

b. Play soothing videotapes for patients. Build a video library that includes tapes of beautiful, restful scenery, travelogues, favorite music, classic films, family or nursing home gatherings, and other personal favorites. Advertise for videotape contributions through your nursing home newsletter.

c. Put up poster-sized pictures of children and grandchildren in residents' rooms with names printed under them. This visual stimulation helps retain personal orientation and keeps memories alive.

d. Encourage families to rotate personal treasures and decorations in the residents' rooms every few weeks.

e. Use hallways and common gathering places as areas for displays of items, such as artworks, beautiful plants, or aquariums.

RECOMMENDATION 4.4   Recommendations for Increasing Visual Stimulation

---

a. Eliminate clutter and keep surfaces clear in personal and common areas.

b. Keep residents' possessions clearly labeled, organized, and separated. Enlist family help in this effort.

RECOMMENDATION 4.5   Recommendations for Decreasing Visual Overstimulation or Clutter

ment of the physical plant (e.g., location of elevators, ice machines and heating or air conditioning vents); (c) the location in the neighborhood (e.g., noisy highways and children's playgrounds); (d) operational factors (e.g., using the television 24 hours a day, recorded background music [Muzak], and noisy paging systems); (e) staff practices (e.g., loud voices and group conversations); and (f) patient disruptions (e.g., crying out, constant moaning, and "sundowning" behaviors). All of these interfere with the residents' abilities to attend, listen, concentrate, and understand. Noise interferes with hearing aid performance and increases ringing in the ears for persons who have tinnitus. It interrupts sleep and increases residents' anxiety, agitation, and irritability. Furthermore, noise begets noise: The noisier the environment, the louder people must speak to be heard (Recommendation 4.6).

2. *Lack of proper amplification where sound and voice need to be heard.* When residents cannot hear important sounds and voices,

a. Use a low-pitched, modulated speaking voice.

b. Monitor the volume of televisions, radios, and paging systems.

c. Encourage all residents to use earphones with their televisions, radios, or audiotapes, especially when roommates have guests or need quiet time.

d. Schedule noisy housekeeping tasks (e.g., vacuuming) when residents are away from the area.

e. *Use sound-absorbing materials to modify hard walls and floors that amplify sound. Carpet floors where possible to subdue unpleasant or loud street and neighborhood noises. Add wall carpeting, throws, drapes, pillows, tablecloths, and plants.

f. *Use sound-absorbing materials around elevators, ventilators, and devices that reverberate, rattle, whine, blow, or have loud on-off mechanisms.

g. *Look for alternatives to institution-wide paging systems (e.g., personal pagers, call systems with quieter bells, and digital systems that allow for hook-up variations.)[4]

*Recommendations that are more likely to cost money or require administrative decisions.

RECOMMENDATION 4.6   Recommendations for Decreasing the Level of Ambient Noise in the Nursing Home

they may be inattentive or may fail to respond. An inability to hear causes embarrassment and leads to isolation, depression, and paranoia (Recommendation 4.7).

3. *Lack of pleasurable or soothing auditory stimulation; lack of familiar sounds and voices.* Human beings find the sounds of music, nature, and familiar voices soothing. When these sounds are missing from the environment, patients miss opportunities for calming interludes and quiet memories (Recommendation 4.8).

Factors Interfering with the Enjoyment of Aromas and Tastes

1. *Lack of pleasant aromas.* An environment that offers few pleasant aromas robs residents of stimulation that stirs their memories about personal sensory experiences. Even worse, unpleasant odors (e.g., from pungent cleaning chemicals, urine and feces, air fresheners and odor "cover-ups," or stale air) discourage visitors, which deprives the residents of opportunities for conversation. The presence of noxious odors also leads to a loss of appetite (Recommendation 4.9).

2. *Lack of positive taste experiences; staff inattention to residents' taste and food preferences; unpleasant dining experiences.*

> **a.** Whenever possible, reduce or eliminate all auditory or visual distractions.
>
> **b.** Train all caregivers, including volunteers and family members, to speak to residents face-to-face at eye level with a low-pitched voice.
>
> **c.** Instruct staff to approach one another when speaking instead of calling across the hall or from room to room.
>
> **d.** Make sure that hearing aids are clean, in good working condition, and have live batteries.
>
> **e.** Outfit your residents' personal tape recorders with earphones to amplify sound, focus attention, and support speech comprehension. Monitor volume control frequently.
>
> **f.** Suggest that families of hearing-impaired patients explore the use of assistive listening devices in the patients' personal areas, especially with Alzheimer's disease patients who can no longer tolerate hearing aids.
>
> **g.** *Install amplification devices on all phones.
>
> *Recommendations that are more likely to cost money or require administrative decisions.

RECOMMENDATION 4.7   Recommendations for Ensuring Adequate Amplification of Sound or Voice

> **a.** Ask family members to bring audiocassettes of "voices from home"—family members (especially grandchildren), pets, favorite hymns, short excerpts from a church or temple service.
>
> **b.** Collect a library of audiocassettes that have soothing sounds of nature, quiet music, the Psalms, or familiar poetry.
>
> **c.** Invite volunteers to be personal readers for those Alzheimer's disease patients who find it calming to listen to a pleasant voice.
>
> **d.** Create and call attention to pleasant homey sounds, e.g., coffee perking, birds singing, children laughing, and church bells ringing.

RECOMMENDATION 4.8   Recommendations for Increasing Pleasurable and Soothing Auditory Stimulation

People will not eat what they do not like to eat. Also, the sense of taste deteriorates with old age. If, in addition, the daily experience of eating is unpleasant, residents are not likely to eat well. You may not be able to improve the quality of food in your facility, but you can try to present it to patients in an appealing manner (Recommendation 4.10).

a. Encourage family members or volunteers to bring pleasant room sprays, fabric deodorizers, colognes, shampoos, and lotions that the patient enjoys and can tolerate.

b. Consider ways to release and call attention to enjoyable aromas, e.g., popcorn, coffee, fresh-baked bread, and cookies, especially just before mealtime. Open the windows for scents of newly cut grass, sea air, or outdoor barbecues.

c. Try not to disinfect residents' rooms just before mealtime.

d. Refer to "Recommendations for Improving Visual Accessibility" to remind patients to use the toilet and thereby avoid the lingering odor of urine.

RECOMMENDATION 4.9   Recommendations for Increasing Positive Aroma Experiences and Decreasing Institutional Odors

a. Use words that describe pleasant aromas and tastes with the residents to heighten their awareness. Invite them to enjoy the different textures and visual aspects of a dish before eating.

b. Insist that feeding assistants know and apply considerate, safe feeding techniques, e.g., avoid large portions of food served too rapidly; be careful not to feed a patient when food is too hot (pureed food especially can be dangerously hot); and alternate flavors, textures, and temperatures with each spoonful. Name the foods frequently.

c. Serve meals "family style" to residents who are still able to eat independently to give them some sense of control over their food choices and to encourage the use of procedural memories.

d. Keep a warmer or microwave oven in the dining area to rewarm food that has grown unappetizingly cold and congealed.

e. Make sure that residents who need feeding assistance receive thorough oral hygiene after every meal (e.g., no remaining bits of food in oral cavity, and lips and fingers clear of food), especially if they are going to lie down within the next hour.

f. Ask family members to bring in favorite dishes or treats that are within the resident's dietary restrictions.

g. Collaborate with dietary staff to vary visual surroundings and presentation of food. Gather ideas from journals, occupational and speech therapists, volunteers, and the resident council on inexpensive ways to develop a pleasant dining atmosphere.

h. Enhance the environment of the dining area or trays with flowers and plants, music, pictures, or bright paper napkins.

RECOMMENDATION 4.10   Recommendations for Increasing Positive Taste Experiences and Decreasing Unpleasant Eating Experiences

**Quick Tip Summary: Environmental Factors
Affecting Communication**

1. Factors interfering with good vision.
   a. Poorly arranged or inadequate lighting; glaring unfiltered light; shiny surfaces.
   b. Lack of visual accessibility.
   c. Missing or inadequate signage and information displays; small, illegible print or too much print.
   d. Too little visual stimulation.
   e. Too much visual stimulation or clutter.
2. Factors interfering with good hearing.
   a. Too much ambient noise.
   b. Lack of proper amplification where sound and voice need to be heard.
   c. Lack of pleasurable or soothing auditory stimulation; lack of familiar sounds and voices.
3. Factors interfering with the enjoyment of aromas and taste.
   a. Lack of pleasant aromas; poor control of odors associated with institutions.
   b. Lack of positive taste experiences; staff inattention to residents' tastes and food preferences; unpleasant dining experiences.

REFERENCES

1. Lawton MP. Environment and Aging. Monterey, CA: Brooks/Cole, 1980.
2. Lawton MP. Sociology and Ecology of Aging: Environment as Communication. In H Ulatowska (ed), The Aging Brain: Communication in the Elderly. San Diego: College-Hill Press, 1985;7.
3. Lubinski R. Environmental Considerations for Elderly Patients. In Dementia and Communication. Philadelphia: BC Decker, 1991;257.
4. Hiatt L. Nursing Home Renovation Designed for Reform. Oxford, England: Butterworth–Heinemann, 1991.

GOOD PRACTICE 4.1   BRAINSTORMING FOR RESOURCES TO IMPROVE THE ENVIRONMENT

Directions. With a small group of your coworkers, carry out the exercises below.

1. What could you and your coworkers do with the following "windfalls" to improve the communication environment of your workplace?

A donation of 50 indoor plants? (25 are in hanging baskets.) _____
_____
_____

A donation of 100 carpet sample squares? _____
_____

Three volunteer hours apiece from each of the following services:
a carpenter _____
_____

a plumber _____
_____

an interior decorator _____
_____

a mason _____
_____

a heating/air conditioning specialist _____
_____

a sign maker _____
_____

a photographer _____
_____

an audiologist _____
_____

2. Select partners and take turns feeding each other *at least five spoonfuls* of applesauce, ice cream, pudding, or yogurt. Discuss these questions:
    a. How did you feel being fed by another person (e.g., out of control; helpless; invaded; pampered)?

    b. How would you describe the physical aspects of the feeder's skill (e.g., rate of food presentation; placement of spoon on your tongue; amount of food on the spoon; position of feeder's body in relation to yours)?

    c. What words, amount of eye contact, gestures, or facial expressions did your feeder use to make the experience pleasant?

    d. Did the experience of being fed affect your desire to eat in any way (e.g., did it seem to affect the taste of the food or your enjoyment of eating)?

    e. As a result of this experience, would you change your approach to feeding residents? How? How would you now advise or supervise others in the procedure?

3. How many patients in your charge would you estimate have a hearing loss?_____. What percentage is this of the total number of residents for whom you care: 25%? 50%? More than 50%? Almost all? Think of one of these hearing impaired residents for whom you care. Find two recommendations from "Factors Interfering with Good Hearing" that you could use to support better communication with this person. (See Recommendations 4.6–4.8.)

GOOD PRACTICE 4.2 FIRST IMPRESSION VISUALIZATION

Directions: Speak slowly and allow participants enough time to develop their imagery. Give the group these instructions:

"We are going to take a guided visualization or mental trip. I will ask you to close your eyes and picture the scene I describe. Afterward, when I ask you to open your eyes, please do not speak until you have written down some important first impressions (pause).

"Now, close your eyes. Imagine that you are a first-time visitor coming to see a friend at the nursing home in which you work. Picture yourself driving into the parking lot. Look around at the buildings and grounds. Walk through the front door. Ask someone how to locate your friend. Find your way down halls and up elevators to the correct room. Pay attention to the sounds and smells that you experience along the way. Notice any sensations you have whenever you touch anything. Observe the personnel and the patients whom you meet—their eye contact, facial expressions, speed of movement, comments to you and to each other. What catches your attention about the decor and the arrangement of the administrative offices, therapy rooms, nursing stations, or patient areas that you pass?

"Now, open your eyes. Please do not speak. Write down the first three impressions that you, as a guest, have just had about the facility in which you work."

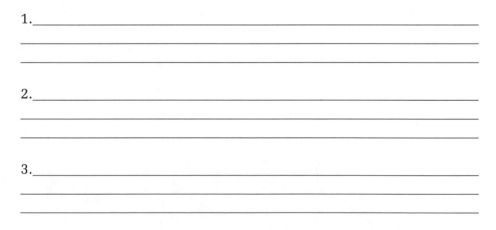

1._____

_____

_____

2._____

_____

_____

3._____

_____

_____

"Good. Now let's discuss and compare impressions."

Effects of the Psychosocial Environment on Communication and Steps for Improving Environmental Factors

UNIT OUTLINE

Premise

1. Often the formal and informal social "rules" of a nursing home can create a psychosocial environment in which residents have little desire or opportunity for communication.
2. Causes and solutions can be sought for psychosocial barriers to communication in the nursing home.

Definitions

Communication-Impaired Environment

Psychosocial Barriers

Overcoming Psychosocial Barriers in the Nursing Home Environment

Factors Interfering with Preservation of Cognitive Functions

1. Too few activities at the Alzheimer's disease patient's level; access to activities is difficult for residents; insufficient transportation to and from activities
2. Lack of awareness of patients' personal history
3. High rate of absenteeism and turnover among nursing home staff

Factors Interfering with Social Interaction

1. Poor arrangement of rooms and furniture
2. Unnecessarily restrictive institutional "rules" or unspoken policies
3. Overuse of impersonal, task-related communication and "ordering"

PREMISE

Although it is unrealistic to assume that lifelong social roles can be completely retained, it is possible to cultivate a social environment that encourages self-sufficiency, independence, contribution, and self-expression to the degree possible for the individual.[1]

Often the formal and informal social "rules" of a nursing home can create a psychosocial environment in which residents have little desire or opportunity for communication. This unit examines the psychosocial factors affecting communication that restrict residents' opportunities for meeting critical cognitive and social needs and offers recommendations for reducing the chances of communication breakdowns.

DEFINITIONS

Communication-Impaired Environment

A communication-impaired environment is one where there are few opportunities for successful, meaningful communication.[1]

Psychosocial Barriers

Psychosocial barriers to communication exist when (a) the environment and the staff members working within that environment do little to support the preserved cognitive and memory abilities of the patient; (b) residents are not socially accepted or treated with respect by staff members or other residents; (c) the basic human needs for privacy and personal space assume low priority in the daily operation of the facility.[1]

OVERCOMING PSYCHOSOCIAL BARRIERS IN THE NURSING HOME ENVIRONMENT

One of the greatest challenges for professional caregivers is striking a balance between meeting the medical and custodial needs of demented patients and satisfying the human social and communicative needs of those patients.

Factors Interfering with Preservation of Cognitive Functions

1. *Too few activities at the Alzheimer's disease patient's level; access to activities is difficult for residents; insufficient transportation to and from activities.* When the remaining cognitive skills of an Alzheimer's disease patient are not maximized and carefully challenged, the patient has less reason to talk and less to talk about. When access to activities is not easily gained, residents will not take the initiative to get themselves going. Isolation, loneliness, and learned helplessness result because of increased dependence on staff members. Communicative-cognitive skills decline rapidly (Recommendation 5.1).

2. *Lack of awareness of patients' personal histories.* Often staff members are unaware of the personal histories of the patients for whom they care or seldom refer to those histories. Staff members also may not take advantage of family members as valuable resources for topics of conversation. Sometimes the cultural preferences and practices of patients are not respected or addressed, e.g., limited or no religious services for minorities, no ethnic holidays observed, and ethnic food prohibited even when a resident has no dietary restrictions. The results can be lowered self-esteem, depression, and depersonalization. Patients are at risk for a more rapid fading of emotional and sensory memories surrounding childhood, family, and regional or national heritage. Staff members also are at risk for the effects of depersonalization, e.g., detachment; indifference; and overzealous attention to tasks, schedules, regulations, and numbers (Recommendation 5.2).

3. *High rate of absenteeism and turnover among nursing home staff.* When the persons with whom patients communicate or bond are not consistently present, patients can harbor a constant feeling of being "left" or abandoned. These feelings lead to confusion, loneliness, isolation, depression, a sense of helplessness, and depersonalization (Recommendation 5.3).

a. Request an in-service training session on adapting activities to your residents with Alzheimer's disease.

b. Ask your supervisor if you can approach committees in your church or community clubs to ask for volunteers who can be trained specifically to transport or assist with Alzheimer's disease patients.

c. Ask family members to list activities that their relatives still enjoy or enjoyed in the past.

d. Look for activities that help residents with Alzheimer's disease to pay attention to and care for others, e.g., care of plants, pets, and other residents.

e. Encourage residents to observe activities even if they do not want to participate. They may be more inclined to join in if they feel less pressure to perform.

f. Subscribe to the philosophy that everything a resident with Alzheimer's disease does all day long has the potential to be a meaningful activity.[2]

RECOMMENDATION 5.1 Recommendations for Providing Accessible Activities at Appropriate Levels for Alzheimer's Disease Patients

a. Complete a "Patient Social Communication Profile" (Good Practice 5.1) on each resident with Alzheimer's disease who is in your care.

b. Ask family members or someone from a similar cultural background to describe to you the cultural practices, traditional foods, and holiday decorations or ceremonies that might have been part of the resident's past. Share the information with your coworkers at staff meetings. Use this personal knowledge in conversations with residents.

c. Consider how this valuable information could be used to maintain even one of the following sensory memories: an audiocassette of Gregorian chants or the Moslem Call to Prayer; a passage from the Jewish marriage ceremony; the aroma and a taste of broth from a favorite dish.

d. Use the memory books (see Unit 12) that family members or activities staff have made with the patients.

RECOMMENDATION 5.2 Recommendations for Appreciating Residents' Personal and Cultural Histories

> **a.** Assemble a photo album of direct care staff members on each shift, both days and weekends. Take head shots for clarity of facial features; print first name below each picture in large block letters with a marker. Peruse the book frequently with residents. Add new photos as new personnel arrive; keep photos in the album for a while after employees leave to remind residents that they have left, e.g., "Oh, there's Sarah. Sarah left to have a baby."
>
> **b.** Provide closure to patients when you go off shift or know you are going to be absent; say good-bye, say that you will return and say when; try to impress on the residents who you are and that you will be thinking of them.
>
> **c.** If you are leaving your job, promise you will try to visit. Leave a memento of yourself.

RECOMMENDATION 5.3   Recommendations for Helping Patients Deal with Absenteeism and Staff Turnover

Factors Interfering with Social Interaction

1. *Poor arrangement of rooms and furniture.* Although the arrangement of rooms and furniture is a characteristic of the physical environment, its effects are felt primarily in the psychosocial realm. The poor arrangement of rooms and furniture can discourage easy interaction with others (e.g., wheelchairs lined up along a wall back to front; chairs placed distantly around the periphery of a room; or side-by-side seating in the dining area or seating across a wide table). Drab decor in common visiting areas can create an uninviting atmosphere. Because communication is not easy for them, patients with Alzheimer's disease are less likely to take initiatives to interact socially with each other. They tend to make more bids for the time and attention of staff members when they cannot see one another or the "goings on" around them. When the environment is coldly institutional, guests are reluctant to come or remain. Visitors and residents alike feel distanced from their conversational partners (Recommendation 5.4).

2. *Unnecessarily restrictive institutional "rules" or unspoken policies.* Nursing home "rules" or unspoken policies often can discourage close friendships, interfere with expressions of intimacy between residents, or dissuade patients from discussing "taboo" topics, such as death, loss of a roommate, deepening medical problems, sex, or depression. Sometimes professional counseling is unavailable to Alzheimer's disease patients. When patients have limited opportunities to express emotion, pent-up feelings are liable to erupt

> **a.** Allow patients to face each other when they are clustered in groups or waiting for services, e.g., hair dresser, podiatrist, physical therapy.
>
> **b.** Arrange furniture in a small circle or conversational group around a coffee table that serves as a focus. Leave space around the table for wheelchairs.
>
> **c.** Strive to make the atmosphere in common visiting areas appear welcome and homey. Encourage staff and family members to contribute to this effort.

RECOMMENDATION 5.4 Recommendations for Arranging Rooms and Furniture to Promote Social Interaction

> **a.** Have the sensitivity and courage to recognize that unnecessarily restrictive practices and taboos exist in your work setting. Regard these taboos and practices as very serious barriers to successful communication with Alzheimer's disease patients.
>
> **b.** Encourage residents to provide emotional support to one another.
>
> **c.** Advocate for programs that help residents and staff members cope with sensitive issues, e.g., spirituality, death and dying, personality clashes, and sexual disinhibitions. Support requests for memorial services; explain the sudden disappearances of roommates rather than tell patients that everything is the same as always, as a parent might tell a child.

RECOMMENDATION 5.5 Recommendations for Overcoming Restrictive Institutional "Rules"

in catastrophic reactions. (See Unit 10 for a definition of catastrophic reactions.) Lowered self-esteem, confusion, and agitation can result (Recommendation 5.5).

3. *Overuse of impersonal, task-related communication and "ordering."* Communication problems are more likely to occur if staff seldom take time for social conversation or quiet companionship. Furthermore, when adult patients are constantly "ordered" or told what to do, they rebel. Incidents of abuse and catastrophic reactions increase as agitation and anger escalate. They feel even more confused, and incidents of learned helplessness increase. Some patients will call out continually because they are not satisfied by the typical staff response (Recommendation 5.6).

---

a. Communicate even if you are too busy to sit down. Chat quietly and casually with the resident while you change sheets, arrange a tray, or comb hair. Talk about your mother, your neighbors, or your dog.

b. Develop several ways of convincing residents to comply (see Units 9 and 10).

c. Increase your use of touch to soften a high rate of task talk and to reduce the resident's sense that all is business and only business.

d. Invite outside acquaintances to volunteer as communication partners to the residents with Alzheimer's disease for whom you care. Lend them this book to use as a guide.

RECOMMENDATION 5.6   Recommendations for Reducing Impersonal, Task-Related Talk and "Ordering"

---

a. Organize a grooming group where residents who can still function at higher levels assist with the grooming needs of residents functioning at lower levels.

b. Enjoin family members and volunteers to assist with combing hair, doing nails, applying make up, and applying pleasant scents.

RECOMMENDATION 5.7   Recommendations for Improving Residents' Personal Appearances and Encouraging Social Interactions

4. *Lack of attention to residents' personal hygiene and appearance.* When residents' personal hygiene and appearance frequently are left unattended (e.g., uncombed hair, dirty fingernails, or unpleasant breath and body odors), potential communication partners are less likely to approach or stay to socialize. In addition to sensory discomfort, patients feel isolation, loneliness, depression, embarrassment, and lowered self-esteem. A resident's poor personal appearance also tends to make family members unhappy with facility policies (Recommendation 5.7).

Factors Interfering with Residents' Rights and Need for Privacy and Personal Space

1. *Lack of private places.* When residents have no access to private areas in which to talk, they lose opportunities for close companionship and intimacy. The personal affairs of the residents and

a. Set aside quiet areas and quiet times. Encourage residents, family members, and volunteers to use these areas in preference to common areas when private conversations are desired. (Perhaps this is an issue for the resident council in your facility.)

b. Place telephones in locations that are accessible yet private.

c. *Install jacks in patients' rooms so that a phone can be brought in, or make cordless phones available to patients. It is much less time consuming to bring a telephone to a patient than to get a patient to the phone. Even those who no longer speak may gain pleasure from hearing familiar voices.

*Recommendations that are more likely to cost money or require administrative decisions.

RECOMMENDATION 5.8   Recommendations for Creating Private Places

a. Refrain from talking about residents in their presence as if they were not there; explain or ask permission before searching through personal belongings.

b. Knock when entering private areas; remember to say "excuse me" when interrupting an activity or conversation; keep residents informed about any procedures being performed, even when you are "sure" they do not understand.

RECOMMENDATION 5.9   Recommendations for Respecting Patients' Rights to Privacy and Personal Space

the families are unprotected from public scrutiny. This leads to frustration, bottled-up emotions, embarrassment, important news left unsaid, and family unease (Recommendation 5.8).

2. *Failure to respect patients' rights to privacy and personal space.* Sometimes staff members or visitors fail to respect residents' rights to privacy and personal space, e.g., failing to knock before entering patients' rooms, talking in front of residents as if they were not there, or not explaining procedures that are being performed. Behaving as if the resident does not exist or has no right to privacy is the ultimate dehumanizing gesture. People deserve to be treated with respect to the end (Recommendation 5.9).

3. *Inadequate procedures for protecting personal property and treasures.* Nursing homes need to be especially vigilant in their protection of a demented individual's personal treasures against theft, breakage, or mysterious disappearances. When an Alzheimer's dis-

> **a.** Frequently review nursing home policy on personal property rights of the patients. Compare your policies with those of other homes.
>
> **b.** Seek the cooperation of family members in bringing in items that are important to the resident but not attractive to others.
>
> **c.** Refrain from overassuring the family that items will be secure, but be extra careful to see that all possessions are secure.
>
> **d.** Refer to the sections on wandering, pilfering, and paranoia in Unit 10 of this book.

RECOMMENDATION 5.10   Recommendations for Protecting the Property of Alzheimer's Disease Patients

ease patient's claim of loss or theft is not taken seriously and addressed, or when residents sense that their personal items are not treated with respect, paranoid and catastrophic reactions escalate. This drains time and energy from an already overloaded staff. Furthermore, when family members notice a careless attitude about their relative's possessions, they are liable to develop a distrust that could lead to a lawsuit (Recommendation 5.10).

Quick Tip Summary: Psychosocial Factors that Interfere with Communication

1. Factors interfering with preservation of cognitive functions.
   a. Many nursing homes have too few activities at the Alzheimer's disease patient's level, or they do not provide sufficient transportation to and from activities.
   b. Staff members are unaware of patient's personal history; staff members do not use the family as a resource, nor do they respect cultural preferences and practices.
   c. The nursing home staff has a high rate of absenteeism or turnover.
2. Factors interfering with social interaction.
   a. The facility's poor arrangement of rooms and furniture discourages easy interaction; the choice of decor is drab and uninviting.
   b. Unnecessarily restrictive institutional "rules" discourage close friendships and intimacy.
   c. Staff members primarily use impersonal, task-related communication with residents or order them around; they seldom take time for social conversation or quiet companionship.
   d. The residents' personal hygiene and appearance are frequently left unattended.

3. Factors interfering with residents' rights and needs for privacy and personal space.
   a. The institution lacks private places for conversation.
   b. Staff members and visitors fail to respect residents' rights to privacy and personal space.
   c. The nursing home has inadequate procedures for protecting residents' personal possessions; claims of loss or theft are not treated seriously.

REFERENCES

1. Lubinski R. Environmental Considerations for Elderly Patients. In R Lubinski (ed), Dementia and Communication. Philadelphia: BC Decker, 1991;257.
2. Hellen C. Alzheimer's Disease Activity-Focused Care. Boston: Butterworth–Heinemann, 1992.

GOOD PRACTICE 5.1   PATIENT SOCIAL COMMUNICATION PROFILE

Directions: Use this questionnaire as a means of orienting staff members to new nursing home residents and as a resource for engaging residents in social communication. The information can be obtained from the patient, the patient's record, or from family members.

1. The decade in which the resident was born; the resident's mother's name:_____

_____

2. The cultural or ethnic background in which the resident was raised:_____

_____

3. The city in which the resident was raised: _____

_____

4. Where the resident went to school:_____

_____

5. Whether the resident is a veteran; during which war; where stationed:_____

_____

6. If married, spouse's name and where married:_____

_____

7. Where the resident lived and worked for most of his or her adult life:_____

_____

8. Resident's occupation; retirement date:_____

_____

9. Children's and grandchildren's names; where they live now:

_____

_____

10. Religious preference:_____

_____

11. Favorite books, movies, or television shows:_____

_____

12. Hobbies, special interests, musical preferences:_____

_____

PART II

Examining Communication Skills of Professional Caregivers

UNIT 6

Communication Strengths and Problems of Professionals Who Care for Patients with Alzheimer's Disease

---

UNIT OUTLINE

Premise
1. Professional caregiving is extremely stressful.
2. One of the primary causes of stress is communication breakdowns between caregivers and Alzheimer's disease patients.
3. These breakdowns may not be solely caused by the person with dementia. Caregivers are at least as likely as members of the general population to have problems that impair their communication skills.
4. This unit examines the communication strengths and weaknesses of persons who care for patients with Alzheimer's disease.

Definition
  Communication Style

Communication Strengths of Professionals Who Care for Alzheimer's Disease Patients

Communication Problems of Professionals Who Care for Alzheimer's Disease Patients
1. Speech, language, voice, and hearing characteristics
2. Gender, status, and age biases
3. Cultural and linguistic differences
4. Personality factors
5. Education and experience
6. Situational influences
7. Responses to the burdens of professional caregiving
   Quick Tip Summary: Communication Problems of Professional Caregivers

PREMISE

Professional caregiving demands enormous amounts of physical, mental, and emotional energy. When your nursing home residents are Alzheimer's disease patients, they offer little cooperation in completing tasks and give few thanks for your efforts. Interactions seem to be discouragingly one-sided. Working with Alzheimer's disease patients has been likened to "being exposed to a severe long-term, chronic stressor."[1] Many professional caregivers find it hard to leave that stress behind when they go home. A comment in a recent study of the effects of caregiving on nursing assistants reflected the feelings of many: "I drive around in my car and cry until I feel like I can go home."[2]

One of the primary causes of the stress is the breakdown in communication between caregivers and the patients for whom they care. Alzheimer's disease patients have multiple deficits that contribute to this breakdown, but the patient accounts for only half of every interaction. The caregiver is the other half. The fact is, the persons in your care may not be the only ones with communication problems. Healthcare workers are at least as likely as members of the general population to have problems that interfere with communication.

This unit will examine the positive and the negative aspects of caregiver communication that are most likely to have an impact on the behavior of patients with Alzheimer's disease. You will assess your own personal communication strengths in working with patients who have Alzheimer's disease and learn about ways to overcome or compensate for your communication weaknesses.

DEFINITION

Communication Style

Your communication style is the set of verbal and nonverbal behaviors that you typically use to send or receive messages. Your personal communication style varies depending on the people involved, the circumstances, and the communication goals for the moment.

> Every day Jack Phillips would put on his coat and tie, ready to go to work as he had done for forty years. We called on nursing assistant Mimi Girard, who knew best how to reason with him. "No, Jack, no work today, breakfast first," she coaxed, "then a shower, okay?" He paused, trying to figure this out, then asked, "Is the car in the garage?" "Yes, Jack," she assured him, "the car is safe and sound."
>
> Somewhat settled, he walked to the day room. Getting him there was more than "assist residents to day room" as listed in the job manual, and coaxing him to take off his coat and tie was more than "give shower." To carry it off took knowing each other and an exchange based on familiarity within partnerships of caretaking.[3]

Illustration 6.1   Adapting Communication to Patient's Needs

For example, a 16-year-old girl may coax the car keys from her father in a childlike way, skillfully shift her style to "mature woman" with her 17-year-old boyfriend, and change again to "silly teenager" with her girlfriends. Seasoned and sensitive caregivers can adapt their communication styles to compensate for the communication deficits of patients with Alzheimer's disease.

COMMUNICATION STRENGTHS OF PROFESSIONALS WHO CARE FOR ALZHEIMER'S DISEASE PATIENTS

Professional caregivers have numerous communication strengths on which to draw that can be used to help Alzheimer's disease patients in their struggle to communicate. For example, when nursing assistants speak and move in a relaxed manner, the behaviors of patients are more flexible, calm, and cooperative. Patients also respond better when assistants use a personal rather than an authoritarian way of speaking. Illustration 6.1 is an example of how one caregiver changed her communication style to meet the particular needs of her patient.

Your work with Alzheimer's patients will go more smoothly and be less stressful when you:

1. Acknowledge your own communication strengths and weaknesses.
2. Are willing to eliminate or change a personal communication style that hinders your work with Alzheimer's disease patients or with others who also care for those patients.
3. Understand the communication losses and retained abilities of patients with Alzheimer's disease.

4. Believe that if you use good communication skills, the patient's cooperation will increase and troublesome behaviors will decrease.
5. Are willing to take responsibility for communicating with an Alzheimer's disease patient.
6. View the patient as an individual with likes and dislikes and a personal history that can be used to reduce confusion or promote compliance.
7. Can recognize and respond quickly to the patient's efforts to communicate.
8. Can adapt your personal communication style to meet each patient's communication needs.
9. Are sensitive to subtle changes in the patient's communication or other behaviors as a crisis-prevention skill.
10. Can maintain a calm communication style during a crisis, especially when the patient is being abusive.
11. Are willing to ask for help in tough communication situations.
12. Are willing to use stress management techniques when your personal tension level becomes too high.

COMMUNICATION PROBLEMS OF PROFESSIONALS WHO CARE FOR ALZHEIMER'S DISEASE PATIENTS

Most of us think that our personal communication styles are more than adequate to get us through everyday situations. We might not be great public speakers, but usually our acquaintances know what we are trying to say. However, a communication style that works well under ordinary circumstances might not be the best one to use when working with Alzheimer's disease patients. Why not? A caregiver's way of speaking can enhance a patient's ability to respond appropriately, but it can also destroy relationships and jeopardize the patient's sense of cooperation and security.

The following seven factors in a caregiver's communication style can significantly impact the communication success of a patient with Alzheimer's disease:

1. *Speech, language, voice, and hearing characteristics.* Every adult exhibits a unique combination of speech, language, and vocal traits that together form a sort of "acoustic fingerprint"—the voice that we recognize on the telephone. Even among normal speakers, some persons mumble or speak in a soft voice; others talk rapidly, have elaborate vocabularies, or use long, complex sentences. Although their friends can follow what they say, these persons would have difficulty communicating effectively with

Alzheimer's disease patients. A caregiver who uses little or no body language, eye contact, or touch is also at a disadvantage in communicating with Alzheimer's disease patients. Persons with Alzheimer's disease rely on the emotional messages of nonverbal communication to function socially, even when they no longer understand speech.

Listening skills also are crucial to successful communication with Alzheimer's disease patients. As patients deteriorate cognitively, their language becomes harder to understand and interpret. Greater effort must be made by the listener to pay attention and listen mindfully; otherwise important information will be missed or misread. Poor listening habits and careless attention to patients' utterances invite an even more rapid decline in their communication skills. Poor listening habits will also create barriers between the caregiver and the patients' families and between the caregiver and coworkers.

Some caregivers have diagnosable communication disorders that go beyond poor communication style. An estimated 10% of all adults have some type of clinical communication disorder—a dysarthria (slurred or unclear speech), a stutter, or perhaps a chronically hoarse voice. Hearing loss is the most prevalent of these communication disorders. The older you are, the more prone you are to loss of hearing. Persons with uncorrected hearing loss may speak in voices that are too soft or too loud for the hearing comfort of others. Their speech may become less precise and more difficult to understand. The reluctance of individuals with hearing loss to ask others to repeat may cause listeners to unfairly judge them as "vague," inattentive, or forgetful. Many of the symptoms of hearing loss are the same as those of early-stage Alzheimer's disease!

Healthcare employees with any of these *uncorrected* communication impairments will have trouble communicating with coworkers, friends, or family, but most especially with patients who have Alzheimer's disease. It is better to do something about the problem than to jeopardize your job and your personal relationships (Recommendation 6.1).

2. *Gender, status, and age biases.* Perceived differences in gender, status, age, and social customs govern the way people speak to each other. We speak more casually with friends and more formally with elders, authorities, or persons to whom we wish to show respect.

American culture is inclined toward negative attitudes about aging and places a high value on youth and beauty. A caregiver who views older, female, or dependent persons as having less worth may be tempted to address them in a patronizing manner, especially if those persons are demented. Any display of bias relating to gender or age will inevitably create serious communication problems on the job.

> **a.** Consult a speech-language pathologist if others often ask you to repeat what you said or accuse you of mumbling. Perhaps a professional can find the cause and help you improve the clarity of your speech.
>
> **b.** Consult a certified audiologist to rule out hearing loss if you frequently must ask others to repeat what they said. Follow the advice of that professional, no matter how insignificant the loss may seem to you.
>
> **c.** Take a course to improve your listening skills if you are often criticized because you have not listened to or remembered important messages. Many good programs are available on audiotape. See also Unit 11 for a definition and explanation of empathetic listening skills.
>
> **d.** Join a community theater group, a poetry reading club, a Toastmasters speaking group, or a Dale Carnegie course if you sense that others miss your meaning because you rarely use nonverbal communication to support your message. Any of these leisure-time activities teach participants to deliver a message with greater impact and confidence. They also serve as excellent antidotes to job stress.

RECOMMENDATION 6.1   Recommendations for Overcoming Your Own Speech, Language, or Hearing Problems

If you persist in speaking to persons of a certain age, gender, or status with less respect, including telling jokes about people with dementia, you will quickly undermine your effectiveness in the nursing home with residents and staff. Everyone responds negatively to an environment in which a toxic speaking style prevails, particularly if they are the targets of such bias (see Unit 9 for a definition of *toxic talk*) (Recommendation 6.2).

3. *Cultural and linguistic differences.* A caregiver's cultural background is one of the strongest influences on communication style. First, there are the obvious differences in pronunciation between persons who speak "standard American English" and individuals who speak a dialect or English as a second language. Accent differences, limited vocabulary, and grammatical errors can cause communication breakdowns among staff members with different linguistic backgrounds, between foreign-born caregivers and Alzheimer's disease patients, or among foreign-born residents from different cultures.

Furthermore, communication styles that are richly rewarded by one culture may raise serious objections in another. In some cultures, people are encouraged to tell stories, show emotion, and assert themselves. In others, the use of broad gestures, direct eye contact, and long speeches would be considered rude. We are all products of our unique upbringing; most of our differences cannot and should not be erased. Nevertheless, they can and should be

a. Know your biases related to gender or age differences. Leave bias jokes and ethnic slurs outside the door of your workplace—or leave the workplace.

b. Avoid using the same trendy language with your elderly patients that you use with your peers.

c. Reject an attitude that suggests "parent-child" or "I'm OK but you don't know what you're doing" when speaking with your Alzheimer's disease patients.

RECOMMENDATION 6.2 Recommendations for Overcoming a Communication Style that Reflects Gender, Status, or Age Biases

a. Understand your own cultural frame of reference and explore the ways it is similar to but different from that of your patients and coworkers.

b. Advocate for diversity training programs in your workplace; attend and learn from them. Cover for coworkers so that they can attend and learn, too.

c. Seek accent improvement if you are having trouble being understood. Tutoring may be found in the speech and hearing or the English as a second language departments of a local college. Sometimes speech-language pathologists offer instruction at group rates; consult the Yellow Pages of your telephone directory.

d. Attend adult education courses in English as a second language or in effective communication. Local high schools and community colleges offer these classes free or at low cost.

RECOMMENDATION 6.3 Recommendations for Overcoming Cultural and Linguistic Differences

studied, appreciated, and accepted by one another within the nursing home community. If cultural differences become the subject of prejudice in your nursing home, effective communication among residents and staff will be at risk (Recommendation 6.3).

4. *Personality factors.* Introversion and extroversion are two personality traits that have definite effects on the communication styles of caregivers. Persons who are introverted may be unwilling to reach out and support communication with a patient with Alzheimer's disease. Extroverted persons may not have the patience to listen with empathy, or they may have a communication style that excites or agitates patients.

a. Assess your personality traits through one of several available means: self-help or Meyers-Briggs workshops, human resources seminars or counseling sessions, or self-help books and questionnaires.

b. Seek "how-to" books, audiotaped courses, classes, or groups that concentrate on improving interpersonal communication. Many weekend or evening workshops specialize in building these skills in a friendly and nonthreatening manner.

c. Keep a journal of your observations and feelings. Keeping a journal is viewed by many experts as one of the most effective ways to work through personal issues, and it is free. Check out books from the library or your church, synagogue, or spiritual community center on how to get the most from writing about your personal journey.

d. Seek professional counseling for persistent or serious depression.

RECOMMENDATION 6.4   Recommendations for Managing Troublesome Personality Factors

Other personality traits, such as tendencies toward denial or depression, feelings of embarrassment or a low tolerance for a patient's deviant behavior, sensitivity to criticism, or an inability to deal with conflict, will negatively influence responses to patients (Recommendation 6.4).

> Staff members who have a quick temper, depression, or extraordinary energy are not appropriate to work with residents with dementia. Assigning the right staff to residents' care whether on or off a unit, can significantly reduce labor costs and certainly improve the quality of life for residents.[4]

5. *Education and experience.* Certified nursing assistants (CNAs) frequently comment that they do not receive enough training in the management of human relationships when working with an Alzheimer's population.[2, 3] Continuing education is vitally important for job performance and job satisfaction. It introduces new terms, techniques, and ideas. It provides a fresh outlook and new motivation to perform better on the job. Unless you enrich your daily experience with continuing education, your enthusiasm will falter and your caregiving style will become ineffective.

Many nursing assistants discover that experience is not always the best teacher. Bad experiences have a way of building barriers to communication. If you care for a patient who has been combative, the fear and hostility that you feel as you approach that person again may show in your body and verbal language. The patient senses

> **a.** Apply and advocate for as much in-service training as possible. Stretch your own educational goals beyond state or federal requirements.
>
> **b.** Stimulate your ideas through professional reading. Professional journals and periodicals are full of information and tips for making your job easier and more satisfying.
>
> **c.** Develop an open mind for bad and good experiences. Good experiences give you confidence; bad ones teach valuable lessons, too. Adopt the attitude: "What did I learn from this that will help me do better or be more effective the next time?"

RECOMMENDATION 6.5   Recommendations for Maximizing Education and Experience

your reaction and responds, not unexpectedly, in a like manner. A vicious cycle of miscommunication begins. Professional caregivers must be resilient and view such experiences as "lessons learned" rather than "getting burned." Trying times will occur, but they should not be more burdensome because of inadequate training and negative experiences. Continuing education should bolster your ability to cope with tough situations and turn them into positive experiences (Recommendation 6.5).

6. *Situational influences.* Many situational factors govern how well a caregiver communicates with Alzheimer's disease patients. You will notice great differences in your communication style and in your patients' responses, depending on whether the setting is public or private, noisy or quiet, task-oriented or social, routine or emotionally charged. For instance, many times the pace of nursing home operations conflicts with the pace of the residents who live in the home. The needs and routines of caregivers and patients seem to exist on different time tracks. Compare the nursing assistant's urgent pleas, "Come on, I haven't got all day!" or "Please, Mrs. Cohen, finish your tray. The girls downstairs are going to pick up soon" with the resident's slow replies, "What did you say, dearie?" or "You're walking too fast. I can't keep up." An awareness of these differences and an ability to adapt your speaking style and your tempo is often crucial for good patient care (Recommendation 6.6).

7. *Responses to the burdens of professional caregiving.* Nursing home employment has many aspects that feel burdensome: absenteeism, understaffing, the limitations of new trainees, double shifts, low pay, heavy physical labor, the demands of recordkeeping and scheduling—the list seems endless. An Alzheimer's disease patient's responses to communication can also become part of the burden. The patients' topics of conversation are not intellectually challeng-

> **a.** Understand how your particular work environment affects communication. Study the environmental factors that have an impact on communication as discussed in Units 4 and 5. Make adjustments so that you and your patients can have the best conditions possible for communicating.
>
> **b.** Guard against letting your choice of words, tone of voice, and body language reflect the exasperation you feel when you are in a hurry and the patient has all the time in the world.

RECOMMENDATION 6.6   Recommendations for Overcoming Situational Factors

ing. Repetitive questions; constant moaning and crying; and confusing, pointless answers may inspire irritation or boredom.

In addition, it is not unusual for professional caregivers to have multiple stresses within their own lives, such as holding two jobs, meeting high medical or school expenses, or caring for their own aging parents. Such constant demands leave little desire or energy for trying to communicate with reluctant Alzheimer's disease patients.

The burdens of caregiving can lead to feelings of helplessness and hopelessness and to an attitude of "What's the use?" Hidden (and not so hidden) feelings of exhaustion, frustration, and resentment begin to show in a caregiver's behavior. Some caregivers stop trying to communicate with patients except when they need to get a job done. Most Alzheimer's disease patients, sensing the caregiver's emotional hardening, respond poorly to this treatment.

Research has revealed that tolerance in caring for patients with Alzheimer's disease is related less to the severity of the patients' problems than to the caregivers' own perception of the burden.[5] In short, how well you respond to your Alzheimer's disease patients depends on how overwhelmed you feel about having to deal with them at all (Recommendation 6.7).

Quick Tip Summary: Communication Problems of Professional Caregivers

Healthcare workers are at least as likely as the general population to have problems and impairments that compromise their communication with Alzheimer's disease patients. These problems may be related to:

1. Speech and language characteristics.
2. Gender, status, and age biases.
3. Cultural and linguistic differences.
4. Personality factors.

> **a.** Cultivate or return to some leisure activities to lessen your stress. Your heart, soul, and body may be crying out for better balance.
>
> **b.** Update your continuing education. Training in new ideas and techniques could give you the coping tools and regeneration you need.
>
> **c.** Seek career counseling if you have a persistent feeling of "What's the use?" about your job. You may need a total change of careers. Or you may do better working with a different type of patient or in a different environment. Decide which path to take and begin to act on your decision right away so that you can feel in control of your life once again.

RECOMMENDATION 6.7 Recommendations for Overcoming the Burdens of Professional Caregiving

5. Education and experience.
6. Situational influences.
7. Response to the burdens of professional caregiving.

A FINAL NOTE ON THE COMMUNICATION PROBLEMS OF PROFESSIONAL CAREGIVERS

The important point to remember is that communication success or failure does not rest entirely with the skill level of Alzheimer's patients alone. Success or failure rests heavily on *your* communication skills as well.

REFERENCES

1. Schulz R, Visintainer P, Williamson GM. Psychiatric and physical morbidity effects of caregiving. J Gerontol Psychol Sci 1990;45:181.
2. Richter J, Bottenberg D, Roberto K. Communication between formal caregivers and individuals with Alzheimer's disease. Am J Alzheimer's Care Rel Dis Res 1993;8:20.
3. Diamond T. Making Gray Gold. Chicago: University of Chicago Press, 1992.
4. Peppard N. Special Needs Dementia Units: Design, Development and Operation. New York: Springer-Verlag, 1991.
5. Zarit S, Orr N, Zarit J. The Hidden Victims of Alzheimer's Disease: Families Under Stress. New York: New York University Press, 1985.

GOOD PRACTICE 6.1 COMMUNICATING WITH OTHERS: WHAT IS MY PERSONAL COMMUNICATION STYLE?

Directions: Take a look at how, when, and under what conditions you communicate most comfortably. Below is a set of 15 questions that probe your typical style of interacting with others. Circle the number of the answer under each question that most closely describes your communication style. Then total all the circled numbers. Use the scale at the end of the questionnaire to interpret your score.

Important! Do not place a value judgment on your personal style of communication. Rather, be aware of your characteristics so that you can adapt them toward more effective interpersonal skills.

A. I like my work environment to be
1. Quiet all the time.
2. Quiet, interrupted by occasional conversation.
3. Generally quiet, but sometimes filled with conversation and music.
4. Generally alive with people and noise interspersed with regular quiet periods.
5. Full of people, activity, and as much music as possible.

B. The number of "social" or "personal" conversations as opposed to business conversations that I have on an average day at work is
1. None.
2. One.
3. Two.
4. Three.
5. Four or more.

C. I consider myself
1. A recluse.
2. Shy.
3. An average communicator.
4. A better-than-average communicator.
5. A "real talker."

D. People tell me that my rate of speech is
1. Very slow.
2. Deliberate.
3. Average, or no comments.
4. Rapid.
5. Too fast.

E. People tell me
1. I talk too softly.
2. I sometimes cannot be heard.

    3. Very little about how loud I am; I must sound normal.
    4. I sometimes talk too loudly.
    5. I speak pretty loudly most of the time.

F. People tell me
    1. They cannot understand my speech.
    2. I often mumble or my accent is "thick."
    3. Very little about my pronunciation; it must be normal.
    4. I am a very good speaker.
    5. I should go on the stage!

G. I would rate my vocabulary as
    1. Limited.
    2. Adequate for daily needs but new words often stump me.
    3. Average; I do all right.
    4. Sophisticated; college graduate level.
    5. Good enough to do the *New York Times* crossword puzzle in ink without a dictionary.

H. My use of body language is
    1. Minimal; I talk with my mouth only.
    2. Infrequent; I sometimes gesture with my hands.
    3. Frequent but limited; I gesture mainly with my hands.
    4. Ample; I use gesture and touch to make a point.
    5. Flourishing; I use all I have to get my message across.

I. The acuteness of my hearing
    1. Is something I've never thought about.
    2. Sometimes seems like a problem, but I've never had it checked.
    3. Has been checked; I could use a hearing aid but do not wear one.
    4. Has been checked; is currently adequate (with or without an aid).
    5. Is excellent; I never miss a thing.

J. My use of humor is
    1. Rare; people tell me I have no sense of humor.
    2. Passive; I enjoy humor, but can't tell a joke.
    3. Occasional; I rely on it once in awhile.
    4. Well developed; I have a good sense of humor.
    5. Constant; I have a great sense of humor, though perhaps I overdo it once in a while.

K. I maintain eye contact during conversation
    1. Rarely; I seldom look people in the eye.
    2. With difficulty; especially with authority figures.
    3. Most of the time with friends and peers, but not with certain people who make me uncomfortable.

4. Fairly easily and fairly often with most people.
5. All of the time; I enjoy "staring people down."

L. I rely on touch when I communicate at work.
1. Seldom; it makes me uncomfortable.
2. Occasionally with close colleagues.
3. Sometimes, when I know the person well.
4. Often, when it seems appropriate to get a message across.
5. Frequently; I consider touch a primary means of communication.

M. I feel responsible for starting the conversation or introducing a new topic
1. Seldom, if ever.
2. Occasionally.
3. About half the time.
4. More often than not.
5. Always, it seems to me.

N. As a listener, I
1. Am primarily a "good ear" and not a talker.
2. Prefer to listen, but talk if I have to.
3. Enjoy listening and responding to what I hear.
4. Prefer to talk, but listen if I have to.
5. Am primarily a talker; I get impatient if I have to listen too long.

O. Relative to my personal communication style,
1. I feel uncomfortable most of the time about the way I speak or sound.
2. I occasionally make errors or have trouble being understood; I wish I could improve.
3. It may not be the best, but I'm not going to change it now.
4. It is adequate, but I'm always looking for ways to improve.
5. It is quite good; I am generally pleased with how I speak and sound.

Score:

60–75: Very extroverted communication style. May need to develop listening skills.

40–59: Outgoing talker. Expectation of leadership role.

20–39: Good listener. May want to develop more speaking initiative.

Below 20: Very introverted communication style. May have difficulty taking responsibility in communication situations.

(Adapted from E Ostuni, MJ Santo Pietro. Getting Through Communicating When Someone You Care for Has Alzheimer's Disease. Vero Beach, FL: Speech Bin, 1991.)

GOOD PRACTICE 6.2   WHAT IS MY PROFESSIONAL CAREGIVER'S COMMUNICATION STYLE?

Directions: Circle the answer that best describes the communication style you use with most of your patients. Take the time to read each of the choices carefully. Discuss your responses with colleagues who have read this unit.

1. When I am with patients, I usually
   a. Don't say much.
   b. Use primarily task talk.*
   c. Mix task talk with social conversation to make the task more pleasant for both of us.

2. When talking with patients, I
   a. Keep moving.
   b. Stand briefly by the patient's bed (chair) occasionally as I work.
   c. Sit down at least once a week and direct my attention solely to that patient for a few moments.

3. I routinely refer to the patients
   a. Always on a first-name basis: "Ida," "Joe"; or as "honey," "sweetie," "good girl," or "naughty boy."
   b. Formally as "Mrs. Jones," "Mr. Smith."
   c. By the name that the patient and family prefer; and with adult praise such as "charming," "endearing," or "nice work."

4. When I need to get an Alzheimer's disease patient to do something, I
   a. Do as much of the task as I can to save the aggravation of trying to explain it.
   b. Tell the patient in no uncertain terms what he or she has to do and that I won't put up with any nonsense.
   c. Get the patient's attention first, then present one instruction at a time and praise the patient for successful completion of each.

5. If patients have low verbal skills, I
   a. Rarely try to communicate.
   b. Say something once in a while just to hear my own voice.
   c. Talk or sing to them frequently and stay alert to any response they make to my communication.

---

*Task talk: A command style of language used to get patients to do something, e.g., "Roll over," "Swallow," "Sit up," or "Move your arm." For further explanation, see Unit 8.

6. When family and friends visit, I
   a. Stay out of the resident's room when visitors are present; avoid family members as much as possible.
   b. Treat family members politely but do not get involved in long conversations.
   c. Get to know family members and observe them with the patient.

7. When I am with patients and coworkers at the same time, I
   a. Don't say much to either.
   b. Talk mainly to my coworker.
   c. Try to include coworker and resident in a conversation.

8. When a coworker needs to talk to me about a confidential matter, and I am with a patient, I
   a. Talk to my coworker as if the patient weren't there.
   b. Leave the resident abruptly to finish the conversation.
   c. Signal to the patient that I must leave but will return shortly.

9. When talking about a patient with Alzheimer's disease to others, I
   a. Don't think it matters what terms I use to describe the resident's behaviors, strengths or weaknesses, or where I am when I say it.
   b. Use only professional terms to describe the patient. That way it doesn't matter to whom I talk or where.
   c. Use positive and professional terms to describe patient behaviors; carefully select to whom and where I speak.

10. The responsibility for helping to maintain the communication skills of Alzheimer's disease patients and making them feel secure and content *through communication* belongs to
    a. Family members, friends, and chaplains, who know the patient the best.
    b. Speech-language pathologists and other therapists who provide special communication treatment and programs.
    c. Every single staff person who comes in contact with the residents, but especially me.

UNIT 7 | Multicultural Issues in Nursing Homes

PREMISE

An individual's cultural background has a profound impact on all aspects of his or her communication. It shapes not only the way that

> Mrs. Fast beckoned to me to come closer so that I could hear her voice, still weak from a recent stroke. "Honey," she rasped, "I think I'm losing my hearing." "What makes you think so?" I asked. Whatever Mrs. Fast's impairments, poor hearing did not seem to be one of them. "I can't understand a word those people are saying." I glanced over at the two aides, a man and a woman chatting cheerfully as they changed Mrs. Fast's bed. They were conversing in Polish.

Illustration 7.1   Challenges of Cultural Diversity

person speaks and sounds, but also how he or she uses gestures and touch, what topics are considered taboo, and how the individual relates to authority. Such communication practices bind people together within a single culture, but they are often a source of serious conflict between people from different cultures.

To meet the growing demands of providing care for the nation's elderly, the nursing home industry hires an increasing number of so-called "minorities" every year. Today, these facilities face the challenges that have been fostered by cultural diversity (Illustration 7.1). Whether the differences are between staff members, between staff members and residents, or within the resident community, diversity issues are best addressed through sensible policies of openness, education, and enrichment.

DEFINITIONS

Culture
Culture consists of the "customary beliefs, social forms, and material traits of a racial, religious, or social group."[1] When we are children, many of the associations that constitute our culture exist within a small circle of people. Later, we may join another religion, move to a different geographic region, and socialize with persons from a variety of backgrounds. Yet even as we stretch to adapt to new surroundings, we retain the stamp of our early cultural beginnings.

Ethnic
Ethnic pertains to "a large group of people classed according to a common racial, national, tribal, religious, linguistic, or cultural origin or background."[1] "Ethnic" is a descriptive term that signifies a particular group and their cultural practices, e.g., the "ethnic food" of Guatemala or the "ethnic dances" of a Native American Indian tribe.

Ethnic is a narrower, more precise term than *culture*. We use *ethnic* when referring to genetic markers and blood relationships as well as when referring to traditional behaviors and beliefs. *Culture* has a broader interpretation and is less strict in suggesting race or parentage. For instance, certain places or groups, such as the Wild West, Cannery Row, Wall Street, or "the homeless," have clear cultural definitions yet include individuals from widely diverse bloodlines. Conversely, we would not talk about the "ethnic food" of Wall Street or the "ethnic dances" of people living in Cannery Row unless we meant to make a joke.

Company Cultures

A good example of how broad the term *culture* has become is the idea of "company cultures." Sociologists note that every organization has a subtle but unique company culture or personality, one that vigorously promotes its own acceptable ways of behaving and speaking.

For example, healthcare professionals must learn a large number of medical terms that are essential for everyday communication in a nursing facility. This vocabulary defines the first level of company culture encountered by nursing home employees. Persons in their first job or who speak English as a second language have to work hard to become as fluent in "medicalese" as their more experienced coworkers.

Apart from the medical vocabulary, every facility has a "lingo" and a culture that gives it a special personality or climate. Employees create words and phrases not used "on the outside." New staff members soon realize that some topics, which are acceptable in other settings, are taboo within the organization. Certain relationships are frowned on; others are encouraged. Humor is often based on "in-jokes" or things that have happened while coworkers were on duty together. The expectation of a company culture is not just that staff members sound "American" or "Chicagoan." They are expected to talk like the rest of the staff does *in this very workplace.* Otherwise, "they" sound "funny." New employees, raised in ethnically different countries or neighborhoods, may find the dual pressure of conforming to American cultural standards and to a particular company culture a heavy burden.

Employees are not the only ones who must adjust to the company culture in a nursing home. The persons experiencing the greatest culture shock on entering institutional life are the new residents. If those residents, uprooted from their previous ways of life or culture, are also disoriented because of Alzheimer's disease, adjustment can be overwhelming in the first days and weeks.

Quick Tip Summary: What Constitutes a Company Culture?

1. The formal or professional language of the workers.
2. The informal or "inside" ways of expression and jokes based on common experiences of the coworkers.

"The nurses from the Philippines were well-trained and highly qualified, but they were from another country and language and this generated some communication gaps. Sometimes they did not understand American colloquial slang and customs.

"Art Loudes, who was 79, sang in his room 'You are My Sunshine' and 'Clementine' with full voice but almost no teeth. To someone not familiar with the song, his singing was only a jumble. Charge Nurse Alvarez, in the United States less than 2 years, took him for demented, made a comment to that effect, and infuriated him to a frenzy. When she realized her mistake, she apologized."[2]

Illustration 7.2   Cultural Differences Between Staff and Residents

3. Explicit and subtle codes of conduct that govern topics and styles of communication, dress, and staff relationships.

IMPACT OF CULTURAL AND ETHNIC ISSUES ON COMMUNICATION IN A NURSING HOME

The effects that cultural and ethnic diversity can have on the lives and relationships of persons who live and work within a nursing home are countless. Staff members need to be aware of how these differences influence communication and how effective communication techniques can help them avoid misunderstandings.

1. *Cultural differences between staff members and residents.* In many nursing homes, a large percentage of the direct care and the support staff members are African-American, Hispanic, or Asian. One New York City home recently reported that its employees represented 84 nationalities. Compare this workforce with a community of residents that is almost all white and primarily of European or North American descent.

When a resident has Alzheimer's disease, the communication barriers are formidable. Cultural differences between staff members and residents created by age, gender, religion, ethnicity, and nationality intensify the problems. Often, staff members and residents share neither cultural bonds nor linguistic codes. Yet the caregiver, spurred by economic and career needs, and the resident, impelled by medical, physical, and emotional needs, must learn to communicate with one another (Illustration 7.2).

2. *Cultural differences among staff members.* Diversity training has been slow to enter the nursing home industry in spite of the

increasing prevalence of culturally diverse staffing patterns. The Hebrew Home for the Aged in Riverdale, New York, developed such a program and gained national attention through an article by I. Fisher entitled "With Care, Nursing Home Bridges Racial Gulf" published in the *New York Times* January 12, 1993: "To the Home's administrators, the program was long overdue, not because racial tension was so bad there, but because they felt that fewer misunderstandings would improve patient care."

Misunderstandings between staff members with diverse cultural histories have the potential to disrupt the quiet routine required by Alzheimer's disease patients. Most caregivers, conscientious in their effort to do a good job, would be surprised to hear that their communication style is a possible cause of problems, yet this can be the case. Each culture thoroughly trains its children in the style of verbal and nonverbal communication that is unique to that society. As adults, these same people may not understand how their choices of words or their tones of voice could negatively affect persons from other cultures. Consider the many ways that cultural "rules" for communication determine the following:

Eye contact
Personal space
Appropriate topics for discussion
Acceptable silence
Laughter, humor
Use of touch
Interrupting
Turn-taking
Opening, closing a conversation
Gender, age, and status roles
Forms of personal address
Celebrations, accepting gifts
Politeness
Customs for dating, courting
Family versus company loyalties

To illustrate, an American-born, English-speaking nursing supervisor might consider the averted eye-gaze of a nursing assistant from a Spanish or Asian culture to be a sign of insolence or inattention. Giggling is an acceptable response in some cultures, yet can be seen as totally inappropriate in the United States. People from different cultures have a strong sense of "personal space"—that is, how near to others they want to be when talking. We Americans prefer about 3 feet between ourselves and our speaking partners. If our conversational partners press closer, we feel invaded ("Get outta my face!"). If our conversational partners move out-

Alice, a 3-year resident of Marymount Nursing Home, was an enthusiastic member of the home's Communication Partners program. Her job was to escort her communication partners to activities. "Good morning, Mr. Levin," she began cheerfully, "I'm here to walk with you to church." "Get outta here," he bellowed, "It's Synagogue, you witch. I go to Synagogue." Both residents withdrew angrily from the Communication Partners program.

Illustration 7.3   Cultural Differences Among Residents

side that 3-foot space, we think they are being distant or trying to end the conversation.

A few other examples: (1) Coworkers in an American nursing home could misinterpret as ungratefulness the practice in many cultures of never opening a gift in front of the giver; (2) Americans are sometimes uncomfortable with a European's openness for discussing personal information, such as age and salary; (3) When a firm handshake, which is prized by Westerners as a sign of personal strength, is met with the loose handshake of someone from an Asian country—"limp" translates to "wimp"; and (4) Professional caregivers from the United States may underestimate the educational backgrounds or skill of persons trained in other countries because they may have difficulty passing English-language examinations.

While the majority group is busy judging others by Western standards, cultural opinion operates in the opposite direction, too. American assertiveness may be seen by foreign-born persons as overbearing; informal manners of speaking and behaving as rude; the day care and "television" method of raising children as shocking. Many people from non–United States cultures do not believe in putting their sick and elderly relatives in institutions. They believe that the family should be the cradle of care. Raised with different values, some employees may be caught between the need for a job and disgust for the American custom that places elderly persons in nursing homes.

3. *Cultural differences among residents.* The residents themselves are not immune to old prejudices and ways of behaving, which are often aggravated by the closeness and routine of institu-

tional living. Many times, their misguided good intentions result in poor communication. When residents quarrel over cultural biases, staff members need tact and understanding to help mend the residents' feelings and prevent future incidents (Illustration 7.3).

Quick Tip Summary: Cultural Diversity in Nursing Homes

1. Effective communication is at risk when people from different cultures work and live together in a closed community.
2. In many nursing facilities, at least 30–40% of the direct care staff consists of persons from different countries, races, and cultural backgrounds. In some homes, the percentage is far greater.
3. In most American nursing facilities, the residents are 90% white, American- or European-born, English-speaking individuals.
4. Finding compatible methods of communication is critical to providing a smoothly functioning environment for residents with Alzheimer's disease (Recommendation 7.1).

Quick Tip Summary: Fostering Good Communication in a Multicultural Setting (Tables 7.1, 7.2, and 7.3.)

1. Learn to pronounce other people's names correctly.
2. Tolerate differences in communication styles if they do not interfere with patient care or harm employee relationships.
3. Observe communication styles used effectively by staff members from other cultures.
4. Trust that others intend to say the right thing.
5. Consider carefully who should counsel a coworker whose communication style is offensive to residents.
6. Support your colleagues' efforts to develop more effective ways of communicating.
7. Support your facility's programs in diversity training.
8. Participate in diversity training with an open mind.
9. Do not assume that communication breakdowns occur only because of cultural or linguistic differences.
10. Do not be overly sensitive about the culturally based slurs of patients with Alzheimer's disease.
11. Look for ways to constantly improve your own communication style.

a. Learn to correctly pronounce the unfamiliar names of persons from foreign countries. Use a person's given name unless he or she offers a nickname. Do not assume that it is okay to "Americanize" a name just because it is easier for you to pronounce.

b. Tolerate differences in communication styles if they do not interfere with patient care or hurt another's feelings. If an individual's way of speaking or behaving puzzles you, do not be too quick to criticize. Tactfully express your interest in learning why they express themselves as they do.

c. Observe others carefully in their care of patients with Alzheimer's disease. Their style of communication, while different, may be very effective. If so, learn by trying to shift your style, not theirs.

d. Trust that others mean to say the right thing even if they do not achieve the best results. Remember that few staff members would jeopardize their jobs by being intentionally rude.

e. Consider carefully who should counsel a coworker whose culturally based communication style, in your opinion, interferes with quality patient care. Which person would the employee listen to and understand best? Perhaps you are the one to speak up. If, however, your fellow employee's communication style seems truly disruptive or if he or she is seriously compromising patient care, then without question, the supervisor is the one to intervene.

f. Show respect for and praise your coworker's sincere efforts to develop more effective ways of communicating. An honest compliment to a peer goes a long way toward establishing a positive communication environment.

g. Support your facility's programs in diversity training. Attend these sessions when they are scheduled. Cover for your coworkers so that they have a chance to attend. Offer your ideas for improvement so that the programs will get better. Advocate for in-service training that concentrates on the diversity issues that exist in your workplace.

h. Participate in diversity training programs with an open mind. White, native-born Americans need to learn about other cultures, both those of nonwhite, native-born Americans and those of people from geographically distant lands. Minority groups should gain a deeper appreciation for the culture, customs, and communication styles of native white Americans, too. Most people find that as they gain greater understanding of their colleagues' backgrounds or their patients' histories, they are able to temper their own negative reactions with more empathy and restraint. Keep this thought in mind: "We cannot change people's race or nationality. Most people would not want to change their religion. The one thing that we all have influence over is our own attitude. . . . What you can do is to try to appreciate this individual and focus on providing quality care in spite of your differences."[3]

RECOMMENDATION 7.1 Recommendations for Fostering Good Communication in a Multicultural Setting

i. Do not assume that when the communication between persons from diverse cultural backgrounds breaks down the miscommunication is always the fault of a non-native who speaks English as a second language. Postpone your suspicions and ask yourself, "Could this disagreement or misunderstanding have occurred even if both persons were from the same place and had spoken the same language all their lives? Is there something else going on here that does not have its roots in cultural differences?" If you happen to be the non-native speaker in question, this "reality check" is an especially good idea. Do not be too quick to blame yourself (or let others blame you) for every misunderstanding.

j. Do not be oversensitive about the culturally inspired insults of patients with dementia. Some patients with Alzheimer's disease have lost the ability to inhibit "rude" statements. Their efforts to communicate are sometimes colored by racial slurs and outdated notions about differences between peoples. They may habitually speak in tones of impatience and irritability.

   If a patient's bitter remarks are directed at you, they can hurt, no matter how much you try to take no offense. Still, arguing with the patient will not change his or her mind. Lashing back with insults only worsens the situation, and you open yourself to suspicions of verbal or psychological abuse (see Unit 8). The cardinal rule is that although you cannot control the patient's offensive remarks, you can control your responses. Your own self-control is what counts most.

k. Finally, no matter who you are or what your cultural upbringing, be on constant lookout for good ideas for refining your personal communication style. Improving personal and professional communication skills should be a continuing education goal for everyone.

RECOMMENDATION 7.1   *continued*

Table 7.1   Communication Styles of African-Americans[4]

Characteristic communication styles	How to apply to everyday communication
Nonverbal	
Generally judge the feelings of others by relying on nonverbal communication.	Do not rely on lengthy verbal accounts.
When listening, tend to look away from person speaking; when speaking, tend to look at the listener.	Do not assume that they are not listening to you if they lose eye contact.
Tend to stand close to people when talking.	Allow the other person to determine personal distance.
Verbal	
Animated, confrontational, and heated interpersonal style.	Expect and accept active style of communication.
Frequent interruptions common in typical conversation.	Accept interruptions as style and not rudeness.
Disagreement often indicated by silence.	Avoid interpreting silence as agreement.
Personal questions perceived as invasion of privacy.	Avoid intrusive or direct questioning style.
A cool attitude often covers true feelings.	Do not accept cool demeanor as reflection of true feelings.
Family and personal problems and relationships not readily discussed with outsiders.	Respect people's right to privacy.

Source: Adapted from E Randall-David. Strategies for Working with Culturally Diverse Communities and Clients. Bethesda, MD: Association for Care of Children's Health, 1989.

REFERENCES

1. Webster's Tenth Collegiate Dictionary. Springfield, MA: Merriam-Webster, 1994.
2. Diamond T. Making Gray Gold. Chicago: University of Chicago Press, 1992.
3. Pillemer K, Hudson B. Ensuring an Abuse-Free Environment: A Learning Program for Nursing Home Staff. Philadelphia: Coalition of Advocates for the Rights of the Infirm Elderly, 1991:57.
4. Randall-David E. Strategies for Working with Culturally Diverse Communities and Clients, Bethesda, MD: Association for Care of Children's Health, 1989.

Table 7.2   Communication Styles of Traditional Hispanics/Latinos

Characteristic communication styles	*How to apply to everyday communication*
Nonverbal	
Tend to stand close to people when talking.	Allow the other person to determine personal distance.
Usually make physical contact in greeting by shaking hands, embracing, or back patting.	Be sure to shake hands when greeting Hispanic/Latino.
Often touch people when speaking.	Avoid pulling away and rejecting friendly gesture.
Eye contact generally avoided when speaking to authority figure. Prolonged eye contact is disrespectful.	Avoid direct or prolonged eye contact. Do not interpret lack of eye contact as inability to relate socially.
Manner of interaction tends to be indirect and low key.	Remember that low key indicates respect and not a lack of feeling.
Latinos expect elders to be treated with utmost respect.	Address elderly Hispanic persons more formally than younger adults.
Verbal	
Many Hispanics continue to have limited use of English.	Find an interpreter to conduct important interactions in Spanish.
Commonly show delays in responding to questions.	Allow time to reply; do not hurry the person.
Do not usually interject, interrupt, or affirm in conversation.	Do not assume that conversation is not being followed when feedback is limited.
Hesitant to share personal or family information with strangers.	Avoid intrusive or direct personal questions.
Hispanics are generally nonconfrontational.	Be sure to establish trust, support, warmth, and caring.
Women are often emotionally expressive, whereas men do little emotional communicating.	Be aware of differences between genders and gauge communication accordingly.

Source: Adapted from E Randall-David. Strategies for Working with Culturally Diverse Communities and Clients. Bethesda, MD: Association for Care of Children's Health, 1989.

Table 7.3   Communication Styles of Traditional Asians

Characteristic communication styles	How to apply to everyday communication
Nonverbal	
Women do not shake hands in traditional cultures.	Do not be the first to extend your hand when meeting an Asian woman for the first time.
Asians consider it inappropriate to be touched by strangers.	Communicate sincerely in a nonphysical manner.
Traditional religions do not allow touching the head.	Do not touch the head of any Asian person, especially an elder.
Direct eye contact is disrespectful.	Establish only fleeting eye contact.
Pointing at people or objects with your toes is considered rude.	Do not cross your legs or stand with one foot on chair, etc., when addressing an Asian.
Waving with palms facing upward can be interpreted as sign of contempt.	Avoid waving.
Smiling or laughing is often used to mask discomfort or avoid conflict.	Do not assume that smiling indicates agreement or pleasure. The opposite might be true.
Emotional restraint is highly valued. Formality and politeness are important.	Avoid being too lively or casual. This might be interpreted as rudeness.
Verbal	
Generally speak in a nonaggressive and self-deprecating style.	Be aware of this cultural style and do not interpret it as low self-esteem.
Often indirect and quiet; nonconfrontational.	If you do not want to offend, do not raise issues that evoke strong feelings or conflicts.
Do not share personal feelings openly.	Respect the privacy of Asians.
Generally defer to others in interactions.	Invite equal participation in conversations.
Often nod and utter words of assent ("I see.") to indicate they are listening.	Do not take words of assent as agreement, necessarily.

Source: Adapted from E Randall-David. Strategies for Working with Culturally Diverse Communities and Clients. Bethesda, MD: Association for Care of Children's Health, 1989.

GOOD PRACTICE 7.1   PAIRED INTERVIEWS

Note: People can work together for long periods (months or years) before feeling comfortable or interested enough to learn about their coworkers' cultural, religious, or ethnic background. This short exercise works best in groups of four to ten persons and can reveal pleasant surprises, even to those who think they know each other well.

Directions: Divide the group into pairs; count off (1-2, 1-2, or apples-oranges, apples-oranges, etc.). Every "1" finds a "2" or every "apple" finds an "orange." Using the following list of questions, have the two persons in each team interview one another. The facilitator should stress *verbal exchange* of information. Participants then use the information about each other to introduce their partners to the rest of the group. Keep the atmosphere informal, friendly, and accepting. Allow ample time for questions and spontaneous conversation at the end. Encourage people to probe for differences in regional and family cultures, not just national and ethnic differences.

1. Name:_____
(Interviewer: Make sure you learn how to pronounce your partner's name correctly!)

2. Where were you born?_____
Where did you spend most of your childhood?_____
_____

3. Tell me about something special you used to do or play as a child, with your family or with neighborhood friends._____
_____

4. Think of one special holiday that your community celebrated. Was special food served on that holiday?_____
_____

5. What view did your childhood community have toward the elderly? How were they treated; how were they cared for if they were sick or frail?_____
_____

6. If you could have one wish in the world, regardless of cost, what would it be?_____

GOOD PRACTICE 7.2 DISCUSSION QUESTIONS ABOUT CULTURAL DIVERSITY

Directions: The following questions, intended for small group discussions, relate to the cultural practices in communication that might arise in the nursing home/health care setting. You may wish to create additional questions that relate to the diverse cultural communication issues in your particular setting.

1. Give some examples of significant gestures used in your culture. Are gestures used lavishly, moderately, or seldom to communicate?
2. How are touch and personal space used in your culture? How is the use of touch related to the status of persons (e.g., parent/child, teacher/student, man/man; and woman/woman, public display versus private). How does distance between speakers depict role, status, and emotion?
3. How is eye contact used in your culture?
4. How important is tone of voice in your language? What are the social rules regarding use of a loud or a soft voice?
5. Describe communication styles that people are expected to use with authority figures.
6. What is the family structure like in your society regarding care for the elderly? What are your culture's expectations regarding home care versus hospital or institutional care? How does your society feel about people who grow "senile"?
7. What are your culture's beliefs and practices about death and dying?

GOOD PRACTICE 7.3   DISCOVERING YOUR COMPANY CULTURE

Directions: Use the following questions for small group discussion.

1. Does your staff have "in-house" words or names for:
    a. Certain safety, medical, or hygiene procedures?_____

    _____

    b. Particular patients or groups of patients?_____

    _____

    c. Specific physicians or administrators?_____

    _____

    d. Certain areas or activities?_____

    _____

    e. Employees who exhibit certain behaviors?_____

    _____

2. Relate at least one joke often told by you and your coworkers as a reference point for humor, trouble, overwork, etc.— a joke that no one outside your workplace would appreciate.

    _____
    _____
    _____
    _____
    _____

3. Compare the cultures of previous settings in which you have worked with your coworkers' descriptions of places where they have been employed (e.g., how easy was it to get to know and be comfortable with your colleagues? Was staff encouraged to work with or against each other? Was it as good on the "inside" as it appeared to be from the "outside"? What was the cultural mix and how did it affect the interactions of staff members and residents?)

    _____
    _____
    _____
    _____
    _____

UNIT 8

Verbal Abuse and Communication Neglect and Their Effects on Communication in Nursing Homes

---

UNIT OUTLINE

Premise
1. The most extreme examples of inappropriate communication are verbal abuse and communication neglect.
2. The prevention of any type of abuse is the responsibility of every nursing home employee.
3. "Toxic talk" is a manner of speaking that has major implications in the spread or prevention of verbal abuse or communication neglect.

Definitions
    Verbal Abuse
    Communication Neglect
    "Toxic Talk" and the Verbally Toxic Workplace

Causes of Verbal Abuse and Communication Neglect
    Quick Tip Summary: Ten Ways to Prevent Verbal Abuse and Communication Neglect

References

Good Practice 8.1 Self-Assessment: Hidden Feelings That Influence Communication: A Group Discussion Activity

Good Practice 8.2 Reporting an Incident of Verbal or Psychological Abuse

Good Practice 8.3 Scenarios for Discussion

> Margaret, a 76-year-old widow with Alzheimer's disease, could never remember if she had eaten a meal. She prowled the unit, foraging food from the tray cart, searching for an occasional stray snack, and begging for additional helpings. The staff worried about her consumption of unauthorized food; they wasted precious time hustling her away from the rooms of other angry residents.
>
> In exasperation, one nursing assistant told Margaret that she would poison the woman's food if she attempted to eat more than she was given. "Maybe she'll stop if we all tell her the same thing," suggested the nursing assistant hopefully.

Illustration 8.1   Verbal Abuse

PREMISE

The most extreme examples of inappropriate or ineffective communication are verbal abuse and communication neglect. Acts of verbal abuse and communication neglect, which experts classify as a form of psychological mistreatment, occur in nursing homes at least four times more often than acts of physical abuse.[1]

The prevention of any type of abuse or neglect is the responsibility of every nursing home employee. This unprofessional and often illegal type of communication is discussed here in the hope that the more you know about verbal abuse and communication neglect, the more effectively you can prevent it. This unit also introduces the term *toxic talk*, a way of speaking that, while not illegal, has major implications for the spread or prevention of verbal abuse and neglect.

DEFINITIONS

Verbal Abuse

Verbal abuse is one of several types of psychological mistreatment in which one person speaks to another with the intention of causing emotional pain. A verbal abuser also attempts to control the other person's behavior through violent words (Illustration 8.1). Some examples are

- Yelling or cursing angrily to scare a patient into action.
- Threatening to throw something at or to hit a patient.
- Threatening to punish a patient if he or she does not follow directions, e.g., "I'll lock you in your room," "No food for a week," or "I'll put rats in your bed."

"We sat tidying up some charts. As I glanced over Mary Karney's vital signs, I remembered the incident when she was crying on the bed and I was told to keep moving. Here were the records of her life signs; they made it clear that formally the nursing assistant's job had nothing to do with talking with Mary. It had, in fact, been more efficient and productive not to do so, the faster to collect the measurements.

"To stay to give Mary Karney an emotional outlet for her trouble was supplanted by the act of taking vitals and moving on. ... Tasks produced numbers that, rather than folded in as part of human relations ... dictated the form of interaction between staff and residents."[2]

Illustration 8.2   Communication Neglect

- Making fun of or playing humiliating practical jokes on a patient.

Communication Neglect

Communication neglect occurs when caregivers avoid looking at, talking to, or touching a patient in ways that suggest deliberate withholding of warmth and nurturing (Illustration 8.2). In some settings, for instance:

- Patients are treated as objects or called by the name of their disorder or prosthesis, e.g., "Go get the diabetic in Room 103"; "Take those wheelchairs down to lunch," (referring to the patients in the wheelchairs).
- Staff concern for efficiency and numbers overshadows the patients' need for comfort and reassurance.
- Tasks are frequently performed in a cold, detached, and dehumanizing way.

When attitudes and practices such as these are the rule rather than the exception, administrative or accrediting agencies may find good cause for investigating the facility for instances of possible psychological abuse.

"Toxic Talk" and the Verbally Toxic Workplace

Toxic talk is an unhealthy form of communication that conveys an attitude of disrespect for a person's humanity, right to privacy, and self-determination. It is a way of speaking to patients that severely undermines a positive communication environment. The intention is not to emotionally harm or coerce, as with verbal abuse, or to ignore, as with communication neglect, but to insinuate that the patient is not worth polite consideration.

> Three staff members from The Manor, just off the night shift, collapsed wearily in the diner booth and watched the waitress pour their coffee. "Anna drove me nuts last night, screaming and yelling," said Miriam, shaking her head. "She's a real pain in the ass all right, but she ain't nothin' compared to her kids. Moaning and bitching all the time," added Sarah. Rita yawned, "How come she's in this dump anyway? Isn't she Mike Penfield's mom, that lawyer guy who's building the big mansion up on Spring Street?"
>
> June, the waitress, finished pouring the coffee. She had a date that night with Anna Penfield's nephew. At a nearby table, two reporters from a local newspaper leaned forward slightly. Their newspaper had built its readership by exposing scandal and abuse in the county's institutions. A member of The Manor's Board of Directors and her husband sat quietly in the booth behind the three employees, scraping up the last of their eggs. Their eyes met.

Illustration 8.3   Toxic Talk

Toxic talk is characterized by a staff member's tone of voice, style of speaking, or careless disclosure of confidential information. Toxic talk may be spoken to or in front of a patient, among staff members, or with outsiders. For example, toxic talk can consist of:

- Using a sarcastic or surly tone of voice or a habitually curt form of speech: "Whatsa matter, ya deaf?" "What? You're wet again? Yuk!"
- Discussing the patient's bad behavior or illness within that person's hearing (even though you are "sure" he or she can no longer understand): "She makes my life miserable with her constant whining." "His doctor says the cancer is everywhere; this guy's a dead duck."
- Talking about a patient in an insulting or otherwise unprofessional manner to other staff members: "He's nothing but a worthless bag of s—." "She doesn't have a brain left in her head." "Uh oh, here comes ol' motor-mouth Mabel."
- Talking about patients by name or other identifying details to persons outside the facility, especially if the remarks are demeaning or reveal confidential information (Illustration 8.3).
- Reprimanding or insulting a coworker or speaking ill of another employee in the presence of patients.

Toxic talk may not be against the law, but it is certainly injurious. It creates a feeling of disrespect for the patients among the staff in that facility. It reflects poorly on the professionalism of the individuals who indulge in it. It undercuts the moral fiber of any work team. It can easily destroy community trust, involvement, and investment. Worst of all, toxic talk reduces caregiver sensitivity and sets the stage for acts of true verbal abuse or communication neglect. Employees at every level of the workforce should guard against the destructive effects of toxic talk.

CAUSES OF VERBAL ABUSE AND COMMUNICATION NEGLECT

In recent years, research on abuse in nursing homes has determined that acts of verbal abuse and communication neglect occur more readily in work settings where:

- State laws and agencies do not provide adequate oversight and protection of the rights of patients with dementia or of their caregivers.
- Managers and administrators fail to create and enforce policies that support caregivers and residents, or that enhance the working conditions and climate of the workplace.
- Personnel are less experienced, especially in crisis prevention and intervention.
- The staff does not receive the proper training in how to prevent verbal abuse and communication neglect.
- Staff members are under work-related stress and are approaching "burn-out."
- Employees have a history of resorting to violence to solve problems.
- Employees harbor negative attitudes toward the patients (e.g., the patients "are like children and need to be disciplined," "will only get worse," or "will never know the difference").
- Staff members are repeatedly provoked by combative or verbally aggressive patients[1, 4, 5] (Illustration 8.4).

Abusive incidents of all types occur more often when the patients are abusive to the staff. A high rate of patient aggression can also be a sign that staff members abusively handle or speak insensitively to the patients on a regular basis. Such treatment tends to escalate into alarming abusive or neglectful incidents.

Recognizing that physical and psychological abuse are chronic problems in long-term care facilities, the Coalition of Advocates for the Rights of the Infirm Elderly (CARIE) developed an abuse prevention curriculum designed specifically for nursing assistants. The program has three major objectives: (a) to increase staff awareness of actual abuse and potentially abusive situations, (b) to equip nursing assistants with appropriate conflict intervention strategies, and

"These patients often are the defenseless targets of long-term care staff who, guided by the belief that a loss of cognitive ability diminishes a person's humanity, dismiss residents with dementia as beyond help and unworthy of care. Other times, patients are victims of staff with criminal records and unchecked violent behavior. ... [However] nearly every expert on the front lines of long-term care agrees that ignorance and exhaustion, more often than malice, are usually to blame in cases where dementia patients suffer."[3]

Illustration 8.4   Staff Predispositions for Abuse and Neglect

thereby (c) to reduce staff-resident conflict and abusive behaviors by staff members.

An eight-module training manual provided text and role-playing opportunities for participants to test various methods of coping with difficult patient care situations. Throughout training, nursing assistants were encouraged to share their own examples of troublesome or provocative patient behavior. The curriculum was tested in 10 nursing homes in the Philadelphia area. Results from the pretest-posttest assessment of 114 nursing assistants were positive: attitudes toward their elderly charges improved, and there was a significant reduction both in patient aggression toward staff members and in the nursing assistants' aggression toward their patients.[6]

Programs such as the one developed by CARIE are meaningful in the prevention of abuse, but they do not constitute the only solution to this complex issue. In nursing homes where abuse, neglect, and an atmosphere supporting or encouraging toxic talk are the norm, the problem is a systemic one that requires the attention and action of facility administrators (Illustration 8.5).

In the final analysis, however, no matter how poor the living and working conditions, such conditions can never justify abusive acts. As a professional caregiver, you must take personal responsibility for your attitudes and the behavior that flows from those attitudes (Recommendation 8.1).

Quick Tip Summary: Ten Ways to Prevent Verbal Abuse and Communication Neglect

1. Value and trust your own experience.
2. Do not allow toxic talk to poison your work setting.
3. Know your limitations; recognize your feelings and how they can affect your work.

"Training is obviously important, but the presumption that the lack of it is responsible for the abuse is a naive conclusion. Caregivers do not learn to be abusive in lieu of proper training necessarily. Their behavior may be the result of chronic stress, pathological influences, inadequate supervision, uninspiring management, environmental conditions, or faulty recruitment and selection procedures.

"Abuse is a human and a systemic problem. … To achieve freedom from abuse, the total context of caregiving must be examined and redesigned."[4]

Illustration 8.5   Systemic Predisposition for Abuse and Neglect

a. Trust your experience. Those of you who are new in the caregiving profession, take heart. The longer you work in your chosen field, the more confident you will feel about staying cool in tough communication situations. With experience, you will begin to realize that the aggressive behavior of patients with Alzheimer's disease is an expression of the disease and not of their personal hostility toward you. This knowledge alone can act as a deterrent against making impulsive or defensive responses.

b. Guard against "toxic talk" in and outside the workplace. When you experience stress at home and then more stress on the job, it is easy to fall into a pattern of sullen responses or an aloof "just doing my job" attitude. This unpleasant manner of communicating is more contagious than the common cold; other staff members and patients are quick to respond in a similar manner. No one expects you to be bubbly and sparkling all day every day, but you can develop a habit of pleasant communication with patients and coworkers. Watch your tone of voice and choose your words with the same care with which you would watch your weight or choose your hair style.

c. Know your own limitations. The caregiver who works with Alzheimer's disease patients every day knows well the feelings that caregiving can arouse. Disgust, contempt, fear, superiority, anger, frustration, and disappointment are but a few of the troublesome emotions you will experience. Yet you and you alone are responsible for your actions. You can and must be in command of your own behavior, especially when you are having trouble managing a patient's behavior. When you feel tensions rising, self-control is the one response on which you should always be able to depend. In tough communication situations, seasoned caregivers learn to stay calm and decide whether to handle the problem directly, to back off and wait a while, or to ask someone else for help.

RECOMMENDATION 8.1   Recommendations for Preventing Verbal Abuse, Communication Neglect, and Toxic Talk

Being aware of your feelings is the first step toward successful control of your own behaviors. Good Practice 8.1 at the end of this unit, entitled "Hidden Feelings that Influence Communication and Behavior," will help you get in touch with your emotions and examine your reactions to them.

d. Establish an informal, personal "buddy system." The buddy system is an excellent way to build teamwork and reduce the occurrence of abusive incidents. Each of us has a different set of "hot buttons." A patient who triggers your emotions may be no problem for your partner; someone who irritates your coworker may be easy for you to handle. If you are caring for a patient who causes particular difficulty, try to arrange with a coworker to help out whenever you are extra tired or frustrated.

Here are two suggestions for making the buddy system work: First, remember to thank your coworker after the crisis is over. You want your colleague to feel like helping you again the next time. Second, be ready to help when your coworker needs you. No, you are not expected to do someone else's job all the time. The buddy system is only a safety net for those rare moments when the behavior of a patient with Alzheimer's disease is too much for one person to handle. Everyone benefits.

e. Observe experienced, skilled coworkers. Learn from one other. Watch carefully when your colleague defuses a situation and note especially the body language and communication that was used to accomplish the task. Refer to the suggestions for dealing with tough communication situations in Unit 10. Use these techniques when you find yourself struggling with a patient and be justifiably proud of your improving skills.

f. Re-read The Resident's Bill of Rights, which, according to a federal mandate, must be posted in every long-term care facility.[7] Ask yourself: "If I were the resident, would I be receiving the kind of care and concern (from me, the caregiver) that I desire and deserve?"

g. Request permission to attend continuing education programs on abuse and neglect. This training can take several forms: classroom or home-study instruction, observation of experienced and skilled coworkers, or a mentoring system within the nursing home. Also, seek out programs that teach effective techniques for working specifically with patients who have Alzheimer's disease. These programs can help you develop mature attitudes about aging and about the needs of an elderly, demented population. You will also learn how to improve the environment in ways that diminish the effects of the Alzheimer's disease patient's frustration and confusion.

h. Know your state's legal definitions of abuse and neglect. Knowledge of abuse laws in your state is central to your professional livelihood. Legal language may be difficult to understand, but should you ever be accused of abuse or neglect, ignorance would not be a legal defense. If you are in doubt about the meaning of the words, find someone who can help.

RECOMMENDATION 8.1   *continued*

i. Know also your state's legal requirements for reporting suspected abuse or neglect and the legal implications of not reporting such incidents. There are federal regulations that protect a so-called "whistle-blower," or person who lets authorities know of a suspected wrong-doing by fellow staff members. For instance, what is your legal protection from job loss or harassment? Are you legally guaranteed continued access to promotions or pay raises? These are questions for which you should have answers before you act.

j. Carefully weigh all the consequences for reporting—or not reporting—suspected abuse. Does your company culture support or suppress an employee's decision to blow the whistle? Might there be an undercurrent of backlash from your coworkers? You should have a sense of whether this option is available and acceptable in your own work situation as well as upheld by the law. That is, you could be correct under the law but still lose your job, be shunned, receive threatening notes, etc.

The decision to make such a report cannot be taken lightly. There are many elements to be considered: the legal, emotional, and financial consequences to you and your family and whether you are willing to shoulder these responsibilities; the safety of the patients; and the emotional climate of the nursing home environment. Remember, too, that even though you are the one who suspects and reports an incident, determination of whether abuse actually occurred will be made by those who conduct the investigation. Finally, you should consider the many consequences of not reporting suspected abuse. Nursing assistants in CARIE training sessions thought of the following possibilities:

- The situation could get worse.
- The patient could be seriously injured.
- The employee could abuse other patients.
- The patient could become ill or die.
- The situation could be discovered by the newspapers.
- If the incident is discovered, you could be legally involved (accessory to the crime).
- You would have it on your conscience.[8]

Perhaps you can think of other possibilities.

Studies from the fields of business and engineering indicate that illegal practices decline where workers know that reporting such incidents is accepted as a fair procedure to deal with the problem. Reporting suspected or known acts of verbal abuse or communication neglect is one way that you might be called on to keep your nursing home abuse-free.

RECOMMENDATION 8.1 *continued*

4. Develop a "buddy system" for dealing with troublesome patients.
5. Observe and learn from more experienced coworkers.
6. Know and uphold your institution's Resident's Bill of Rights.[7]
7. Attend continuing education programs on prevention of abuse and neglect.
8. Be familiar with the legal definitions of abuse and neglect in your state.
9. Know your obligations and rights regarding the reporting of incidents of suspected abuse and neglect.
10. Carefully weigh the consequences of reporting—or not reporting—suspected incidents of abuse or neglect in your institution.

REFERENCES

1. Pillemer K, Bachman-Prehn R. Helping and hurting. Predictors of maltreatment of patients in nursing homes. Res Aging 1991;13:74.
2. Diamond T. Making Gray Gold. Chicago: University of Chicago Press, 1992;159.
3. Foote J. Dementia: abuse and neglect compound the suffering of many elderly. Newark (NJ) Sunday Star Ledger, May 7, 1995; Section one(Middlesex ed):1.
4. MacNamara RD. Freedom from Abuse in Organized Care Settings for the Elderly and Handicapped: Lessons from Human Service Administration. Springfield, IL: Thomas, 1988;71.
5. Tellis-Nayak V. Nursing Exemplars of Quality. The Paths to Excellence in Quality Nursing Homes. Springfield, IL: Thomas, 1988;131.
6. Pillemer K, Hudson B. Model abuse prevention program for nursing assistants. Gerontologist 1993;33:128.
7. U.S. Congress. Resident's Bill of Rights. Omnibus Budget Reconciliation Act, 1987: Nursing Home Reform Act. Public Law 100-203.
8. Coalition of Advocates for the Rights of the Infirm Elderly. Ensuring an Abuse-Free Environment. Philadelphia: Coalition of Advocates for the Rights of the Infirm Elderly, 1991;73.

GOOD PRACTICE 8.1   SELF-ASSESSMENT: HIDDEN FEELINGS THAT INFLUENCE COMMUNICATION: A GROUP DISCUSSION ACTIVITY

Directions: In Part I, write in (a) the patient's name, (b) the patient's behavior (repetitive moaning, incontinence, etc.), (c) your feelings (rage, disappointment, inadequacy, etc.), (d) how you are tempted to react (throw a plate, quit, curse, cry, etc.). In Part II, write in possible causes and professionally acceptable solutions. Discuss your answers with the group and brainstorm for further ideas about causes and solutions.

Part I

When patient (a: write patient's first name or initials) _____
does or behaves like (b: describe the resident's behavior)_____

_____

I feel (c: describe your emotional reaction)_____

_____

_____

and I'd like to (d: describe how you would *like* to react)_____

_____

_____

Part II

One reason the behavior might be occurring:_____

_____

One part of my behavior that I might change; one new thing in my approach that I might try:_____

_____

One change in the environment that might help:_____

_____

_____

One other person who might be helpful and in what way:_____

_____

_____

GOOD PRACTICE 8.2   REPORTING AN INCIDENT OF VERBAL OR PSYCHOLOGICAL ABUSE

Directions: In the following decision tree, report the incident only if all answers to the questions are "yes."

Today's Date:_____ Date of Incident:_____

1. Describe the incident as clearly as you can:_____
   _____
   _____
   _____
   _____

2. Did you actually see or clearly overhear the incident?   Yes/No

3. Can you identify the patient involved?   Yes/No

4. Can you identify the staff member involved?   Yes/No

5. Are you able to clearly describe the incident?   Yes/No

6. Do you believe that it was the staff workers' intent to hurt the patient emotionally or physically?   Yes/No

7. Do you believe you are doing the right thing by reporting the incident?   Yes/No

---

GOOD PRACTICE 8.3   SCENARIOS FOR DISCUSSION

Directions: Choose at least two scenarios from the following selection or compose original scenarios based on events that have occurred in your nursing home. Break the group into teams of two or three persons each using the selected scenerios. Ask each team to answer the following five questions; then reassemble the group for general discussion.

Discussion Questions:

1. Does this scene depict verbal abuse, communication neglect, or toxic talk? Why or why not?
2. Making a judgment on some incidents is not so easy; you may be unaware of certain "extenuating" circumstances. If your group is in doubt about how to judge a scenario, try to work out the possibilities by completing this statement: "It depends on whether_____. If this is so, then it probably is_____. If that is so, then it probably is not_____."
3. If the situation seems to be a case of verbal abuse or neglect, what are some possible ways to resolve the problem?
4. If the scene does not seem to be abuse or neglect, are there any ways the situation could be improved to benefit the patient or the caregiver?
5. Has anyone in this group ever witnessed or experienced a similar situation? What was the outcome? Does your group think this outcome was fair, or correct?

Scenario 1: Max has a habit of accosting visitors to his unit and asking for cigarettes. He is very aggressive, peering myopically at the surprised guests and holding onto their sleeves. When Agnes is on duty, she steers him firmly into his room and sits him down in a chair. "It's very rude to ask strangers for anything. Don't leave this room until I say you can." Then she closes the door firmly. Max has arthritis in his hands and cannot open the door easily by himself. He is terrified of being in a closed room by himself.

Scenario 2: George, a certified nursing assistant, was having a hard time getting Julius washed up. Julius flailed and thrashed about and sometimes George's jaw or shin was in the way. Finally, in frustration George yelled: "Stand still, dammit."

George's loud voice and stern face startled Julius and for a moment he stood meekly while George scrubbed away. Then he began to thrash and protest again. This time, George's voice boomed, "Sonovabitch! You stand still or you're gonna have soap in your eyes—in your mouth—up your ass; I'll make sure of it."

Scenario 3: Angelica helped 82-year-old Mathilde into her room. Wordlessly, she undressed the old lady, slid a nightgown around the thin body, and guided her into bed. She took Mathilde's vitals, charted the results, and switched off the light. Before leaving the room, she turned with her face in the shadows and asked the still figure on the bed, "Do you want a glass of water before I leave?" Mathilde, who had poor vision and hearing, returned her gaze but said nothing. Angelica shrugged and left the room.

Scenario 4: It was 2 AM and Evan's voice echoed endlessly down the hallway: "Mother—mother! I gotta go to the bathroom." The words were slurred, but as often as Stewart and Marie had heard them, they had no trouble figuring out what the old man was yelling. Marie complained: "That guy's voice is driving me crazy, like fingers on a blackboard. Can't anything shut him up?" Stewart looked up from his clipboard. "Aw, what's the use? He's on his way out anyway. Besides, when he's gone, we'll just get another screamer. They dump all the worst ones onto this unit."

Scenario 5: Seventy-eight-year-old Renata was admitted to the nursing home while she recovered from hip surgery. A short time later, she was diagnosed with Alzheimer's disease. Her family and the nursing staff also suspected that she was losing her hearing. Renata was not an easy patient to care for. If she did not like someone—and she did not seem to care for most people—she spit or scratched when the individual drew close to her. Nursing assistant Doris and was one of the few staff members who could get Renata to cooperate. "Come on, you crazy old coot," she would croon in her low-pitched voice. "I'm gonna get your butt out of bed if it kills me. I never saw such an ugly puss. Get that foot on the floor before I belt you one." Then she would get right up into Renata's face. "Don't you look at me like that. You spit at me, I'll spit right back. One big hocker for another. You'll be sorry." She would often declare laughingly to the rest of the staff: "I know how to handle her. She doesn't know what I'm saying anyway." The others, relieved that they did not have the job, were willing to agree.

Scenario 6: Joe lay helplessly in his bed, his body and mind almost spent from the ravages of Alzheimer's disease. A few staff members stood at the nurses' station charting the last bits of patient information before going home for the night. "I heard he was a real hell-raiser in his day. Mama told me about all the women in town he screwed," mused Suzanne. "It wasn't just girls from what I heard," added Eric with a cynical tone of voice. "When he was more alert, I made sure I knew where his hands were." Rose, just 2 days into the job and only 1 week away from graduation, listened wide-eyed and wide-eared. Today, when she was changing Joe's sheets, his hands had seemed to "wander" even though his eyes were closed. She sure didn't want that dirty old man feeling her up.

Scenario 7: "Time for lunch." Helen's voice and touch to Madge's back caused Madge to startle and look up. "I always make Madge jump that way if I really want her to do something. If I come at her face to face, she just ignores me."

Scenario 8: Beside the bed: "Get your pants on. Not that way. Here, this way. God, you're stupid. Finally got 'em on? Let's go." Walking down the hall: "Family's waiting. Got ants in their pants. Hurry up. They haven't got all day, neither do I." In the elevator: "Wait'll I tell 'em how bad you've been this week. They'll never wanna see you again. D'ya think they really care anyway?" Entering the reception area: "Here he is at last. Sorry he looks so goofy. Had a hard time getting him dressed again."

Scenario 9: Guests were shocked to hear the way Vera spoke to Nat, who sat slumped over in his wheelchair. She squatted low on the floor so that she could see his face and called in a loud low-pitched voice, "Nat, wake up. Time for lunch." He stirred as she tapped his arm. "I'm putting a pillow under your elbow. Sit straight. Good." Her voice carried down the hall. "Heads up, we're on our way." As they approached Nat's dining room table, she moved around to the front of the wheelchair and blared to a more erect and alert Nat: "Looking good, Nat. Have a nice lunch." He nodded in acknowledgment.

"I'm glad I don't live here," shuddered the visitor to her husband. They had come to the nursing home to see his convalescent brother. "I sure would hate to have someone yell at me all the time like that."

Scenario 10: "Nursie, when's breakfast?" whined Pete. The nursing supervisor rolled her eyes at Pete and sighed. "Twenty minutes, Pete, 20 more minutes. Go to your room and wait." In less than 5 minutes, Pete was back. "Nursie, breakfast. When is it? I'm hungry." The supervisor was talking to Patricia. She didn't like to be interrupted. "Fifteen minutes, Pete. I'm busy now." In a few minutes, there he was again. The supervisor was writing and when he asked the same question, she didn't look up. Pete approached two other staff members near the desk, but no one noticed.

Breakfast finally arrived. Pete was one of the first ones to receive his tray because for a while at least it kept him quiet. About 10 minutes after the trays were cleared, Pete limped up to the nurses station once again. "Nursie, when is lunch?" If anyone heard him, they didn't show it.

PART III

Building Communication Skills with Patients and Families

UNIT 9

Positive Techniques for Successful Conversation with Alzheimer's Disease Patients

---

UNIT OUTLINE

Premise

1. Conversation is a natural therapeutic technique.
2. Given the right support, many patients with Alzheimer's disease are still capable of brief, meaningful conversations.
3. The attempts of Alzheimer's disease patients to communicate deserve to be treated with respect.
4. Fewer abusive incidents or catastrophic reactions are reported in work settings in which caregivers are generous in their use of social communication with patients. (See Unit 10 for a definition of catastrophic reactions.)

Definitions

Conversation
Task Talk
Institutional Talk
Social Conversation
Conversational Success

Talking with Alzheimer's Disease Patients: Four Conversational Techniques That Work

1. Choice question
2. Matching comment/association
3. Closure
4. Repair

Talking with Alzheimer's Disease Patients: Two Techniques That Do Not Work

1. Direct order
2. Affirmations

Quick Tip Summary: Techniques for Successful Conversations with Alzheimer's Disease Patients

References
Good Practice 9.1 Identifying Conversational Techniques
Good Practice 9.2 Four Sample Conversational Scripts

PREMISE

No one has ever found a better therapeutic technique than conversation. Alzheimer's disease patients often are so impaired that any social conversation with them is difficult and may seem useless. "What can I say? He's not going to answer anyway." "He doesn't make any sense." "She can't understand me, so why try?" Why indeed?

First, given the right support, many patients with Alzheimer's disease are still capable of having brief but meaningful conversations. These opportunities to maintain social abilities should not be lost. To keep patients in the "conversation game," you must encourage them to communicate to the best of their abilities whenever and however that can be done. Second, in spite of massive impairments, the patients' attempts to communicate deserve to be treated with respect. Caregivers who respond to a patient's efforts in a positive manner do much to protect the patient from feelings of worthlessness and despair.

Third, fewer abusive incidents or catastrophic reactions are reported in work settings where caregivers provide liberal amounts of social communication along with the necessary task-oriented communication. Alzheimer's disease patients tend to be less disruptive when their social as well as their medical and custodial needs are met. This unit describes a number of techniques that can help you develop successful conversations with your Alzheimer's disease patients.

DEFINITIONS

Conversation

A conversation is two or more people talking to one another on a subject of mutual interest. It is only one avenue of communication, but it is the one with which we are most familiar.

Task Talk

Task talk is the type of communication that caregivers use to get patients to do something. The underlying agenda is to maintain efficient caregiving. "Turn over now." "Here's your lunch. Sit up." "Move your arm." The language is basic and functional. The tone of voice may be warm and friendly, but task talk works best if it is short and uncluttered by detail, especially with an Alzheimer's disease patient. Studies show that at least 67% of all talk directed to nursing home residents by caregivers is task-oriented.[1] The disadvantage of task talk is that it limits the patient's incentive to practice social conversation skills. Task talk invites patients to respond in one of two ways: complain or comply. As important as task talk is for getting a job done, if used to excess it casts the patient into a passive role and fosters dependency and learned helplessness.

Institutional Talk

Institutional talk is a style of communication defined by attitude and tone of voice. The speaker's voice or words come across as false and exaggerated, as when humoring a small child. The underlying agenda is to maintain a parent-child relationship. Institutional talk uses "we" and "our" instead of "you" and "I", as in "It's time for our medicine." Take, for example, the voice of a staff person gushing loudly over the patient's pureed diet: "Look at those delicious carrots! Better eat them all. Our cook will feel real bad if you don't. My, don't we love that smell!" Institutional talk is meant to be friendly, teasing, and cheerful, but actually it distances the caregiver from the patient.

Like task talk, institutional talk discourages two-way conversation. Most people, even those with dementia, feel bored, embarrassed, and demeaned when they have to endure institutional talk. Because Alzheimer's disease patients can sense emotional intent and body language long after they cease to understand words, institutional talk does little to raise their self-esteem.

Social Conversation

Through social conversation, we establish relationships and nourish self-esteem. The underlying agenda is to maintain adult-to-adult communication. "Bella, how's your sister?" "We saw the best movie last night!" "Where did you get your hair cut? I love it." As the abilities of persons with Alzheimer's disease decline, the language of caregivers often becomes stereotypic and dull. Caregivers stop sharing tidbits from their personal lives; they no longer look for new topics to interest their patients. Their interactions become solely task talk or institutional talk. Patients, however, will seldom make an effort to respond genuinely to anything except social conversation.

Conversational Success

Conversational success is true interaction, spoken between adults, lasting for as little as 5 seconds. It does not depend on eloquent speech or serious subject matter. What counts is that two people have shared or connected with each other for a moment. Conver-

Anita, a volunteer at Merryhart Nursing home, was distressed by Maude's insistence that the two women once were neighbors. Every time she passed Maude's wheelchair, Maude reminded her of events and people they once knew. Then to Anita's embarrassment, Maude would scold her about not coming to visit more often, complaining and crying all the while. Protested Anita, "I was never her neighbor! I never heard of any of those people. I try to tell her that but she won't listen." "Does it matter so much that Maude is mistaken about who you are?" chided the nursing supervisor gently, "We're just so pleased that she wants to talk to you."

Illustration 9.1   What Is Conversational Success?

sational success with an Alzheimer's disease patient is achieved through support of the patient's efforts to function as a sociable human being. You will be more successful in your conversations with an Alzheimer's patient if you:

1. Watch carefully for signs that the patient wishes to communicate.
2. Accept responsibility for keeping the conversation alive by using helpful prompts and phrases.
3. Introduce topics that the patient enjoys and that are at his or her level of understanding.
4. Accept even brief exchanges as being worthwhile.
5. Stop worrying about the "correctness" or "logic" of the patient's utterances.

During the next few hours on your job, pay attention to how many instances of task talk, institutional talk, and social conversation you use with your patients:

1. Is more than half of your talk with patients task-oriented?
2. How often do you hear yourself speaking in institutional talk?
3. How many true social conversations do you have or attempt to have with your patients?

Bohling[2] found that when eight human service workers in an adult day-care center conversed with clients, the workers seldom attempted to listen or speak in the frame of reference of the Alzheimer's disease patients. In general, they spoke only of their own interests and did not listen to the patients. The patients with Alzheimer's disease expressed frustration with caregivers who controlled the conversations and ignored their attempts to join in (Illustration 9.1).

TALKING WITH ALZHEIMER'S DISEASE PATIENTS: FOUR CONVERSATIONAL TECHNIQUES THAT WORK

Four techniques that are helpful in conversing more successfully with Alzheimer's disease patients are choice questions, matching comments, closure, and repair. There is no special magic about these techniques. We use each of these techniques every day to keep our conversations going, but research has shown that these four techniques are especially powerful in helping Alzheimer's disease patients stay with a conversation.[3]

1. *Choice question.* A choice question is a request phrased so that the listener has a choice between two things, e.g., objects, words, or opinions. When you use a choice question, you put two pieces of information before the patient on the chance that he or she will recognize the best choice and feel encouraged to make a response: "Elsa, were you married in Scranton or Pittsburgh?" "Harry, would you rather wear the blue shirt or the one with brown stripes?"

When stuck for an answer, people do better with "recognition" than with "recall" types of questions.[4] For example, an anatomy quiz that has open-ended questions such as "To which system does the small intestine belong?" seems more difficult than a test that has a choice of possible answers: "The small intestine is part of (a) the respiratory system, or (b) the digestive system?" In a true/false or recognition-type test, even students who have not studied have a 50% chance of getting the correct answer.

The "recognition" theory also works with Alzheimer's disease patients. Questions that are too open-ended or nonspecific may not offer enough information to an Alzheimer's disease patient about how to respond (e.g., "What did you do today?" or "Tell me about your children"). Alzheimer's disease patients are unable to give the elaborative answers that most open-ended questions require, so they say nothing. Conversation finished. When talking with an Alzheimer's disease patient, you will have more success with conversational moments if you use choice questions instead of open-ended questions.

Questions that can be answered with a simple "yes" or "no" can also stop conversation (e.g., "Did you have a good time?" "Have you met Hannah's new boyfriend?" "Do you want some more ice cream?"). Alzheimer's disease patients tend to respond in the shortest, easiest way possible. Yes/no questions allow them to answer without making any effort to add information. Stay away from yes/no questions if you want to experience conversational success.

2. *Matching comment/association.* A matching comment or an association is a technique in which you offer your own opinion or some information about your personal experience. This natural technique is effective with some Alzheimer's disease patients. If the patient muses "I love red roses," you could reply, "You love red roses? My favorite flowers are pansies. I plant pansies every spring." The resident might be inspired to respond, "Roses—lotsa work," or "Spring is for pansies," or even, "I had a garden."

3. *Closure.* Closure is used when the last word or two is omitted from a sentence in order to let the listener "fill in the blanks." Closure is another nice way of avoiding yes/no questions. "Let me see," you might say, "Your daughter's name is—?" Some patients will not notice the cue, but even severely impaired Alzheimer's disease patients sometimes respond when the ritual is a familiar one or when real objects are used. For instance, you might gesture with the coffee pot and say, "How about a cup of—?" The more a word is used, the longer it remains available to the patient.

4. *Repair.* A repair is a word or statement that corrects the patient's utterance or fills in a missing piece of information. A repair allows you to correct the patient's mistakes without insulting the person or discouraging a rare attempt to communicate. For example, the patient says, "Boy, is it snowing!" Instead of replying, "No, Josh, that's rain. It's raining, see?" you could make a repair by saying, "Yes, it's pouring rain. I really got wet from that rain this morning." With a repair, you affirm the resident's desire to communicate and you correct and/or add information. Though brief, the exchange becomes a successful conversation instead of an instructional "put-down."

A repair is also made when a specific word is substituted for some vague term used by the patient. Opportunities to try the technique of repair are frequent because Alzheimer's disease patients use so many "fuzzy," nonspecific words, such as "it," "that thing," "over there," and "the other one." This kind of language is referred to as "empty speech" because it seems to lack meaning (see also Unit 2). Empty speech is so characteristic of Alzheimer's disease that listeners tend to dismiss it as merely confusing and unimportant. However, if you observe the context closely and think about the patient's personal history, you can often interpret a statement and make a successful repair.

Listen for words that do not carry much meaning, then fill in the words you think your patient meant. For example, if the person says, "It's over there," you might repair by answering, "Yes, your robe is in the closet." If you have guessed incorrectly, the patient may even correct you. For example, you may say, "James, I understand you grew up in Cleveland." James may respond, "Pittsburgh."

> **a.** Do not argue when you and the patient have opposite goals.
>
> **b.** Use words that describe or affirm the patient's behavior. For example, the patient tries to leave but you have not finished dressing her. You might say, "Feeling pretty restless today, hmm?"
>
> **c.** Redirect the patient's attention to another activity or topic. For example, "Let's walk for a moment. My, look at that snow! Remember those winters when we were kids?" After a few steps or a few moments of chatting, the patient may be persuaded to resume dressing.

RECOMMENDATION 9.1   Recommendations for Avoiding Direct Orders

In this instance, the patient has repaired your speech! In any case, your conscious use of the repair technique has succeeded in increasing the Alzheimer's disease patient's active participation in the conversation.

TALKING WITH ALZHEIMER'S DISEASE PATIENTS: TWO TECHNIQUES THAT DO *NOT* WORK

1. *Direct order.* Many times, a caregiver wants a patient to do one thing, while the patient is determined to do another. In this situation, the caregiver might instinctively respond with a direct order. For instance, while you are putting on her house slippers, the patient stands up abruptly and prepares to leave. You say, "Sit down. I'm not finished." Direct orders are all too often ineffective. The patient leaves anyway, and you feel unsuccessful and frustrated.

Research has shown that the more commanding or demanding a caregiver is, the more resistant persons with dementia become.[5] Like all human beings, Alzheimer's disease patients become defensive when they are ordered about. A direct order is neither the best way to build a patient's self-esteem nor a good technique for maintaining social conversation skills (Recommendation 9.1). (See Unit 10 for more suggestions on coping with resistance and refusal.)

Direct orders are not the same as task talk. Task talk does not need to be commanding to be effective. You can give instructions in a pleasing tone of voice, softened with reassurance, sprinkled with praise, and personalized by using the individual's name. Direct orders, on the other hand, are "bossy" in tone and intention. The

> **a.** Use affirmations only occasionally by themselves.
>
> **b.** Use affirmations in combination with requests or directives to soften the impact and to reassure the patient that all is going well. For example, the patient keeps pulling his foot away and complaining. You might say, "I know, I know, you don't like to have your toenails clipped. OK, please let me hold your foot. Um-hmm. That's it. Almost done with your toenails. Good job."

RECOMMENDATION 9.2   Recommendations for Using Affirmations

more you improve your other communication skills, the less often you will need to resort to direct orders.

2. *Affirmations.* Affirmations are short responses such as "Yes," "Um-hum," "I know," and "Oh." As listeners, we use affirmations to show interest in what our companions are saying and to keep them talking. However, to stay on topic, persons with dementia need to hear many concrete words—words that remind them of the names of things. They need encouragement, and affirmations alone are not encouragement enough. Like open-ended questions, repeated affirmations do not carry enough information to help Alzheimer's disease patients develop responses. Conversation quickly dies (Recommendation 9.2).

Quick Tip Summary: Techniques For Successful Conversations With Alzheimer's Disease Patients
Use:

1. Choice question: a question that contains the word "or" and gives the person two choices.
2. Matching comment or association: a response that draws from the caregiver's personal experience or opinion.
3. Closure: an unfinished sentence that the patient is encouraged to complete.
4. Repair: a word or statement that corrects the patient's error, fills in missing information, or replaces a vague term with a concrete one.

Avoid:

1. Direct order: meeting a patient's resistance with a command. (More effective: describe or affirm the patient's feelings, actions, or words, then redirect the behavior.)

2. Affirmations: brief, agreeable responses that do not give enough information to help the patient think of an answer. (More effective: use affirmations to encourage and to soften requests or instructions.)

REFERENCES

1. Seers C. Talking to the elderly and its relevance to care. Nurs Times 1986;82:51.
2. Bohling H. Communication with Alzheimer's patients: an analysis of caregiver listening patterns. Int J Aging Hum Dev 1991;33:249.
3. Santo Pietro MJ, DiCotiis E, McCarthy JM, Ostuni E. Conversations in Alzheimer's disease: implications of semantic and pragmatic breakdowns. Paper presented to the annual convention of the American Speech-Language-Hearing Association. Seattle, WA, 1990.
4. Wilson B, Moffat N. Clinical Management of Memory Problems. Rockwell, MD: Aspen, 1984.
5. Hamel M, Gold D, Andres D, et al. Predictors of consequences of aggressive behavior by community-based dementia patients. Gerontologist 1990;30:206.

GOOD PRACTICE 9.1   IDENTIFYING CONVERSATIONAL TECHNIQUES

Directions: Write down the conversational techniques that the staff member is using in each example (i.e., choice question, matching comment, closure, repair, direct order, or affirmations). Then circle "E" or "I" to indicate whether the techniques is usually "effective" or "ineffective" for fostering social conversation with Alzheimer's disease patients.

1. How about some more—(showing patient a piece of pie).
    _____ E/I

2. We have a guitar player coming. Would you like to stay in your room or go hear the music?_____ E/I

3. You're from Ireland? The necklace I'm wearing came from Ireland. _____ E/I

4. Oh. Um-hum. That's so. I know. Well.
    _____ E/I

5. Patient says: "Cold out. I need a coal." You reply, "Yes, it is cold. Wear the blue coat. You need a coat."
    _____ E/I

6. Sit down right now._____ E/I

7. You're right, Pete. It's a sunny day. The kind of day I like to work in my garden._____ E/I

8. So your daughter is visiting. Is this Marissa or Claire?
    _____ E/I

9. Hurry up, finish this. _____ E/I

10. Patient says, "I want that thing." You say, "Here's your wallet, the wallet with your pictures in it."
    _____ E/I

GOOD PRACTICE 9.2 FOUR SAMPLE CONVERSATIONAL SCRIPTS

Directions: The following pages contain excerpts from actual conversations that occurred between Alzheimer's disease patients and their conversational partners.

Script 1

In this example, the conversational partner repeats many nouns to help the patient develop the topic. The patient was very soft-spoken and never initiated conversation on her own. But if her partner took her to a quiet corner with no distractions, the patient still showed an amazing ability to converse.

Near the end of the conversation, the patient could not think of the word for "spring." Once her partner used the label however, the patient recognized it and used it in her next response. This is a good example of how a repair (supplying the noun for the vague term) effectively supports further replies from the patient.

Circle every noun (names of things) that the communication partner uses. Circle every noun that the patient uses. Compare the totals. Notice that the patient would have used even fewer nouns had the partner not used repairs.

Read this successful conversation aloud with one of your colleagues. How long did it take you to read the entire exchange? (seconds or minutes?)_____

Conversational Partner: "Seeing that shirt you have on makes me—."

Patient: (Interrupting) "Isn't it? It's too much though. I think it's too gaudy."

Conversational Partner: "I think the colors and the flowers are lovely."

Patient: "I had it hanging in the closet and thought I'd better wear it."

Conversational Partner: "I see one flower there that really makes me think of spring."

Patient: "This one. The lilac."

Conversational Partner: "I thought I saw a daffodil right there. See?"

Patient: "A daffodil? Oh, yes, that's right."

Conversational Partner: "Daffodils are one of the first flowers of spring. Right after the crocuses."

Patient: "Right. I've noticed one thing out, the crocuses. They're popping up right now, aren't they, the crocuses?"

Conversational Partner: "Yes, the crocuses are popping up now."

Patient: "I thought so because it's almost time for it."

Conversational Partner: "Um, it's almost time for spring."

Patient: "Spring, right."

Script 2

In this example, the patient is at a later stage of the disease. Look for and label the four effective conversational techniques: choice, closure, matching comment, and repair.

The patient's partner missed a good opportunity to make a repair near the end of the conversation when the patient said, "They're all gone." How could the conversational partner have replied?

Your suggestion for repair: _____

_____

_____

Patient: (Sneezes)

Conversational Partner: "God bless you!"

Patient: "God bless *you!*"

Conversational Partner: "It sounds like you have a cold today."

Patient: "I do."

Conversational Partner: "This cold weather makes colds come. But today is lovely. Look at that beautiful blue sky. Is it clear or cloudy?"

Patient: "What?"

Conversational Partner: "Joe, is it clear or cloudy outside?"

Patient: "It's nice. It's clear."

Conversational Partner: (Looking at Joe's name tag) "Let me see your name tag. Your name is—?"

Patient: "Joseph."

Conversational Partner: "Some people are named after their relatives. What about you?"

Patient: (Nods head) "I was named for my grandfather."

Conversational Partner: (Pause)

Patient: "Our children are gone."

Conversational Partner: "Your children—?"

Patient: "They're all gone."

Conversational Partner: "They're all gone. Oh, that happens."

Patient: "Yeah. Tomorrow or the next day they're coming away."

Conversational Partner: "Your children are coming to see you?"

Patient: "Next day or two."

Script 3

This script is a good example of how the communication partner avoided getting into a power struggle to keep the patient in the room. The conversational partner used choice questions, described and affirmed the patient's impulsive behavior, then redirected him gently with her conversation. *Look for and label each choice question and description of the patient's behavior.*

Compose your own repair to the patient's last comment: "Yeah, they try to fix it up." What clearer verb than "fix" could you use when talking about treating a cold? Also, what words would you suggest to replace "they" and "it"?_____

_____

_____

Conversational Partner: "Do you want to sit, or stand up again?"

Patient: (Stands up)

Conversational Partner: "OK, it feels better when you stand up."

Patient: "Yeah."

Conversational Partner: "Should I stand up next to you or sit down?"

Patient: "I don't care. I want to go back."

Conversational Partner: "We can stay right here. That's not a problem."

Patient: "No?"

Conversational Partner: "No. Let's listen to some music. I hear some big band music out there."

Patient: "My head's warm."

Conversational Partner: "Yes, it's a little bit warm. I don't think you have a fever. Do you need to go to the doctor?"

Patient: "I don't like doctors. No."

Conversational Partner: "No, you'd rather stay home and take care of yourself."

Patient: "Yeah, they try to fix it up."

Script 4

This conversation demonstrates how even our best efforts are not always successful. Although the patient seemed to recognize the topic, she was probably being asked to process more information than most Alzheimer's disease patients can handle.

If her communication partner had described her behavior and empathized with her restlessness, the patient's attention might have returned. And then again, it might not! If each communication moment is an opportunity for the patient, it is also a challenge for the staff member.

Write a different response to the patient's remark: "I can't finish this." Use words that describe or affirm her behavior._____

_____

_____

_____

Conversational Partner: "I watched a TV show last night about a large ship that sank in the ocean a long time ago. The ship was called the Titanic."

Patient: "Oh, I remember that."

Conversational Partner: "You do?"

Patient: "Yeah."

Conversational Partner: "Lots of people were on the Titanic."

Patient: (Indicating her cake) "I can't finish this."

Conversational Partner: "Oh, just put it there and you can have more later. You said you remembered the Titanic?"

Patient: "Um hum."

Conversational Partner: "You remembered it being a big ship? A big ship?"

Patient: "Yes. I can't finish this."

Conversational Partner: "That's OK. You can put it right down there. The Titanic hit a big iceberg."

Patient: "I can't finish the tea either."

Conversational Partner: "You can just sit with it. The Titanic hit a big hunk of ice. The ship rocked back and forth."

Patient: "And it sank."

Conversational Partner: "It sank. I don't think many people survived."

Patient: "Right. I'm gonna go back."

UNIT 10

Positive Techniques for Handling Difficult Communication Situations with Alzheimer's Disease Patients

---

UNIT OUTLINE

Premise
1. Even experienced caregivers find it difficult to communicate effectively with an Alzheimer's disease patient who is acting out or who exhibits a chronic irritating behavior.
2. Staff members need reliable communication techniques to prevent or ease catastrophic situations when they occur.
3. Staff members also need to know how to turn a patient's annoying, repetitive behaviors into moments of positive interaction.

Definitions
    Catastrophic Reactions
    Irritating or Repetitive Behaviors

Communicating Effectively When Coping with Catastrophic Reactions

Communicating Effectively When Coping with Chronic or Repetitive Behaviors
1. Hallucinations
2. Repetitive requests or statements
3. Resistance or refusal
4. Wandering and pilfering
5. Paranoia
6. Severe dementia
    Quick Tip Summary: Difficult Communication Situations

References

Good Practice 10.1 Difficult Communication Situations: What Would You Do?

PREMISE

Pillemer and Bachman-Prehn have noted: "Although new staff receive training on the technical aspects of providing care, they generally receive no training in ways to handle interpersonal problems that arise with patients."[1]

Even the most experienced caregiver finds it difficult to communicate effectively with an Alzheimer's disease patient who is having a catastrophic reaction or who is offering more than the usual amount of resistance. Professional caregivers also find it wearisome to offer supportive communication when their patients display irritating chronic behaviors that are characteristic of Alzheimer's disease. Staff members need reliable communication techniques to prevent such behaviors and to ease difficult situations when they occur. The techniques described in this unit should make your job easier and help you accomplish your care, safety, and treatment goals more quickly.

DEFINITIONS

Catastrophic Reactions

Patients with Alzheimer's disease sometimes respond in an emotional way that seems inappropriate or out of proportion to the situation. Such emotional outbursts, known as catastrophic reactions, reflect the patient's inability to cope with real or imagined events. The reaction may be triggered by an event in the present or by one from the distant past. Communication breakdowns between patients and caregivers often occur during these critical moments.

Irritating or Repetitive Behaviors

Communication with Alzheimer's patients is also difficult when they persist with irritating behaviors associated with dementia (i.e., hallucinations, repetitive verbal behaviors, resistance and refusal, wandering and pilfering, and paranoia).

COMMUNICATING EFFECTIVELY WHEN COPING WITH CATASTROPHIC REACTIONS

Caregivers selected to work with Alzheimer's disease patients are usually given special training in coping with catastrophic reactions. In essence, this unit redefines these same coping techniques in terms of effective communication (Recommendation 10.1). The goals are:

a. Arrange a set of signals with other staff members to be used when you need help. Do this before a critical moment arises. If you wait until a crisis occurs and then have to yell or scramble for help, you risk startling the patient into further panic.

b. Eliminate distractions, e.g., blaring television, people moving around, or lights glaring. This step is essential if you want to get and hold the patient's attention.

c. Notice the body language and tone of voice of the patient. What emotions are being transmitted: fear, anger, frustration, confusion, or sadness?

d. Use the communication techniques suggested below to avoid triggering the patient's physically defensive reaction:

  1. Be aware of your own body language; move slowly, keep your arms down and hands open.

  2. Establish eye contact as much as possible. Keep your facial expression open, warm, and friendly.

  3. Use a reassuring or guiding touch, but only if you think the resident can tolerate touch at this time.

  4. Speak slowly in a calm, firm, low-pitched voice. Remember that you are speaking to an adult, not a child. Take care not to sound sing-song or patronizing; avoid sounding too parental or overly "jolly."

  5. Use the person's name as an alerting cue; use your own name as orientation: "John. It's me, Nancy."

  6. Provide frequent reassurance: "I'm here to help you."

  7. Speak in short sentences.

  8. Try humming or singing softly to distract or soothe.

RECOMMENDATION 10.1   Recommendations for Using Effective Communication When Coping with Catastrophic Reactions

- To keep the situation from escalating.
- To accomplish the task at hand safely and efficiently.
- To return the patient to expected routine.
- To understand the meaning of the patient's message.

COMMUNICATING EFFECTIVELY WHEN COPING WITH CHRONIC OR REPETITIVE BEHAVIORS

Let us now look at six chronic behaviors that are typical of patients with Alzheimer's disease and at the communication techniques professional caregivers might use to cope with them more successfully. Your goals in dealing with chronic or repetitive behaviors include:

- Reducing staff and patient frustration.
- Understanding the patient's underlying message.
- Reshaping repetitive behaviors into useful communication.
- Reshaping staff responses to the patient's behavior.

1. *Hallucinations.* If the patient is having hallucinations but is not upsetting or harming others, consider using the occasion to create a "conversational success" (for a definition of conversational success, see Unit 9). You can be attentive but noncommittal, neither denying nor agreeing with the patient's statements. By listening carefully, you may learn something important about the person. This information could be useful later on.

If the individual is frightened by the hallucination or is upsetting others, refer to the communication techniques suggested for catastrophic reactions. Above all, provide verbal reassurance: "I can help you," or "I'm right here with you." If possible, gently guide the patient to another topic, activity, or location. Keep an object in your pocket that has an interesting texture, color, or scent (for example, a pretty scarf) to encourage a shift in focus. Try music, audiocassettes of nature sounds, or visually soothing videotapes of beautiful scenery to create a different set of images for the person. Do not waste time and energy arguing with the patient about whether the perceptions are "real" or "true."

2. *Repetitive requests or statements.* A common verbal symptom of persons with Alzheimer's disease is the frequent repetition of questions, requests, or statements. To gain a clearer idea of how best to respond to the patient's needs, first try to understand why the behavior is occurring. There are at least two possible reasons for repetitions.

First, repetition can result from memory problems. Alzheimer's disease patients have overwhelming memory problems. One way to reduce repetition caused by memory problems is to address the memory deficit itself. Many patients retain an ability to read and understand single words until late in the disease. You can capitalize on this preserved ability by using single words, short phrases, or visual aids, such as familiar pictures, to stimulate memories. Several studies of nursing home patients have indicated that this technique has much potential for patients with Alzheimer's disease.[2]

Here is a suggestion that is an adaptation of one of these techniques. Suppose you have a resident who continually asks when lunch will be ready. Using a regular manila folder and a black marker, print a short list of words that explain the day's activities. Put the words in a column and use lower-case letters. You may even illustrate each word with simple line drawings (Figure 10.1). Give this "Daily Schedule" to the patient to carry around. This provides caregivers and patients with a common *visual* focus. Each time the patient asks about lunch, a staff member or volunteer points to the

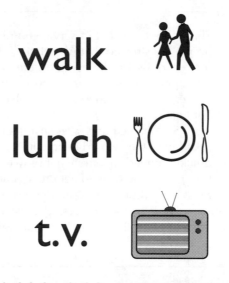

Figure 10.1 Simplified daily schedule of patient's activities.

words on the folder and says: "Harvey. Look at your schedule," and points to the correct answer.[2] Some patients with Alzheimer's disease learn to refer independently to their memory devices. Others become quiet for longer periods of time because they have their own folder. The memory book, described in Unit 12's section on direct intervention programs, may also prove helpful in reducing annoying, repetitive verbal behaviors.[2]

Second, repetition can result from loneliness or boredom. A patient who makes constant bids for attention soon begins to annoy a busy staff. The last thing caregivers feel they are able to do is to stop and talk. Furthermore, caregivers might question how 1 or 2 minutes of "one-sided conversation" could change the patient's repetitive behavior. Yet if every coworker on that shift agreed to spend an occasional moment of companionship with that patient, the cumulative time spent might have a significant impact on the person's loneliness or boredom. The more formalized Communication Partners program, described in Unit 12, is another method for easing a patient's sense of isolation in an organized and ongoing way. In that program, volunteers or fellow patients are recruited and trained to be regular communication companions with Alzheimer's disease patients. Keep one thing in mind, however. Volunteer programs such as Communication Partners, although effective, do not free professional caregivers from their communication responsibilities. Alzheimer's disease patients often feel more secure talking with familiar staff. The importance of your accessibility and the comfort of your personal attention should never be underestimated.

Throughout a recent in-service training session at a large nursing home, we stressed that Alzheimer's disease patients, even more than the rest of us, dislike being ordered about and resist this communication approach strenuously. Several alternative communication techniques were explained and modeled. Then it was time for practical application.

Staff participants were given a tough communication situation and asked how they would handle it. A nursing assistant in the first row quickly replied, "Here's what I say to this one patient that I take care of. 'Mr. Jones, you have to get dressed now. The minister is coming and you must have your clothes on. Put those pants on, **now**!'"

Later, this same nursing assistant complained: "Mr. Jones never does what I tell him to." Without realizing it, she had illustrated our point perfectly.

Illustration 10.1   Effects of Resistance and Refusal

3. *Resistance or refusal.* There are at least three typical reasons why refusal and resistance occur. The primary reason is that patients with Alzheimer's disease find it exceptionally irritating to be ordered around.[3] Second, the patients may not understand what is expected of them. Finally, for Alzheimer's disease patients, any change, however small, means going from the known to the unknown. Change represents fearful insecurity. Their instinctive response is to resist (Illustration 10.1, Recommendation 10.2).

4. *Wandering and pilfering.* Wandering and pilfering are characteristic of many persons who have impaired memory, cognition, and perception. When an Alzheimer's disease patient wanders into other patients' rooms and takes their possessions, fellow patients become frustrated and angry. They feel their private territory has been invaded—and it has.

Institutional environments and routines often intensify the problem of wandering and pilfering. Alzheimer's disease patients become confused when all doorways look alike, when nameplates with small print are placed above eye level, and when their seats in the dining hall have no familiar identification. Constant changes in roommates, staff, visitors, volunteers, and physicians add more confusion. Patients with Alzheimer's disease have difficulty remembering the names and roles of all these people.

It may be impossible to reason with a wandering or rummaging patient who has Alzheimer's disease. Instead, try looking at the problem from a different point of view. Sometimes the way we label people and behaviors influences the way we manage them. Consider renaming the behaviors, reshaping staff responses, and rearranging

a. Begin the task in a quiet spot; if you are in a noisy environment, reduce visual and auditory distractions before giving directions.

b. Speak to the person at eye level. Standing over the patient suggests that you are "boss" or "parent." If a patient feels as if he or she is being treated like a child, his or her responses are more likely to be dependent and childlike.

c. Learn to phrase directions so that your words enlist the patient's cooperation rather than demand compliance. See Unit 9 for further suggestions.

d. Use words of reassurance frequently.

e. Combine verbal with nonverbal directions, e.g., "Please move your foot." Then point to or touch the person's foot.

f. Rephrase rather than repeat your words exactly. Saying the same thing in different words sometimes helps an Alzheimer's disease patient understand.

g. Simplify and shorten your requests.

h. Give only one direction at a time.

i. Say the same key words over and over to remind the patient of the task.

j. Use a firm voice but one that is quiet and friendly. When your communication style is brusque and demanding, the patient is liable to become more fearful and resistant.

k. Keep your goals small and flexible so that you and your patient can delight in many small accomplishments rather than fume over one big failure.

RECOMMENDATION 10.2 Recommendations for Effective Communication When Patients Resist or Refuse to Cooperate

the environment so that finding one's way is easier, and "inappropriate" behaviors can be seen as acceptable (Recommendation 10.3).

When caregivers develop thoughtful solutions to problems that arise with patients who wander and pilfer, they are also protecting the security and privacy of the facility. This is not a small issue for families or security inspectors.

5. *Paranoia.* Another behavior that is characteristic of Alzheimer's disease patients is paranoia—that is, the belief that someone is trying to steal from or hurt them in some way. As a professional caregiver, you understand that the patient's suspiciousness is usually the result of brain deterioration. It is easier for you to be objective than it is for the unsuspecting fellow resident who has just been accused by an Alzheimer's disease patient of stealing from or plotting to kill him or her. That individual is more likely to react with predictable hurt or anger. How do you avoid a heated argument? Think of the Alzheimer's disease patient's paranoia as a deep-

a. Place room nameplates, printed in large, black, lower-case letters, at the patients' eye level. Place some other personal or distinguishing mark by each door to orient the patient. Use this familiar identification on any place or object that the patient is expected to occupy or use: e.g., dining room location, chair on deck, or craft project. Give each Alzheimer's disease patient a laminated room card that matches the distinguishing mark described above. Attach to the resident's clothing with elastic banding. Guide the patient by matching the laminated room card to the name plate.

b. Personalize patients' rooms with unique names, such as "Rose's Garden Room" or "Anita's Arbor." Hotel and restaurant owners learned long ago that customers are attracted and soothed by labels that set a pleasant tone. This type of creative, easy, and inexpensive "de-institutionalization" is more appealing to visitors, too.

c. Develop more appealing terms for wandering or intrusive behavior, such as "shopping" or "sight-seeing." Other patients may be a little more tolerant of the label, if not the behavior.

d. Find other socially acceptable solutions, e.g., community cabinets where patients are welcome to rummage to their hearts' content; or a "shopping" area where patients are allowed to pick up anything they like, such as "sight-seeing" materials, videos, and "tours" to more appropriate locations.

RECOMMENDATION 10.3   Recommendations for Coping with Wandering and Pilfering by Alzheimer's Disease Patients

seated fear that his or her most valuable possessions (cognition, memory, health) are disappearing. Without these, the individual feels extremely vulnerable to harm. This frame of reference will help you choose your words and actions with greater wisdom and caring (Recommendation 10.4).

Although patients with Alzheimer's disease are well known for their paranoid suspicions, this does not mean that they are never victims. Their complaints often go unheeded or misunderstood because people do not take them seriously. How does your facility reassure Alzheimer's disease patients and their families that personal safety and possessions are protected? Are your measures sufficient?

6. *Severe dementia.* Caregivers need their most creative communication skills with patients who are in the final stages of dementia. Table 10.1 describes the communication characteristics of severely demented patients and the effect that severe impairment has on the communication of caregivers. Crying out or disruptive vocalization is one of the most disturbing of these behaviors.

a. Make restoring order your first goal. This is not the time to get caught up in an argument about who is right or wrong.

b. Be a mediator—that is, respond with equal sensitivity to both parties involved. For example, if Alice has accused Joe of stealing her rosary, you might say, "Joe, I know you feel angry." and then, "Alice, you don't like being without your rosary, do you?"

c. Be a communication model. One or both persons might begin to imitate your controlled tone of voice and calm down.

d. Lead the accusing patient away to a quiet area as quickly as possible, and talk comfortingly about the safety and protection of the nursing home. "We're here to take care of you, Alice. We'll help you find your rosary."

e. Return soon to the accused patient. He or she deserves reassurance too. Praise the person for any restraint or tact that was shown during the incident, e.g., "Joe, I was very impressed with your patience today." Your praise may encourage that person to react calmly in future incidents.

RECOMMENDATION 10.4   Recommendations for Coping with an Alzheimer's Disease Patient's Paranoid Accusations

Disruptive vocalization can take many forms: loud or repetitive verbal utterances, nonsensical sounds, screaming, moaning, and constant requests for attention.[4] There are at least three explanations for the continuous stream of cries that are made by some late-stage Alzheimer's disease patients: (1) they may be sick or in pain, (2) they may be responding to some indefinable or uncomfortable sensory experience and calling out is the only way left for them to get help, or (3) the cries may be the body's last effort to find stimulation or release. Whatever the reason, the noise constitutes a major environmental management problem.

As Table 10.1 illustrates, the problems that constant crying out create are not endured by the patient alone. The staff's communication styles are deeply affected by the disruption. Continual moaning raises the noise level of a facility and increases stress on staff. People talk louder and turn up their radios and televisions. Patients who cry out distract other patients and interrupt their rest. To many visitors and potential consumers, such wailing typifies the institutional atmosphere of a nursing home. Without a doubt, this situation affects the communication performance of everyone in the facility. Crying out is a late-stage neurologic response that can no longer be reshaped into useful communication. Instead, your goal must be to reshape the environment and your response to the behavior.

Table 10.1   Characteristics of Communication in Severely Demented Patients and Typical Ineffective Caregiver Responses

Characteristic	Caregivers' ineffective communication responses
Patient is mute, has palilalia, or constantly cries out.	Caregivers may isolate patient physically; talk, work over the noise; cease attempts to communicate socially with the patient; may be less sensitive to cries as genuine requests for help or signals of pain or illness.
Patient is no longer able to draw or use information from the environment or from other persons because of severe perceptual and cognitive impairments.	Caregivers may become careless in speaking about the patient, his or her condition, or other confidential information. May make less effort to appeal to the senses of touch, smell, or vocal intonations to carry messages that do not rely on words.
Patient has great difficulty ambulating or operating wheelchair or is bedridden.	Caregivers may be less inclined to make activities available to the patient or to leave normal routines and work paths to say "hello."
Patient may have rare "windows of lucidity," i.e., understands and responds fully for a moment to the situation.	Caregivers may interpret these incidents to mean that the patient "really understands more than he or she lets on," or that the patient's inability to respond at other times is "stubbornness" or "resistance."
Patient does not self-feed, is at risk for dysphagia because of memory or sensory deficits.	Caregivers may not take precautions against aspiration; may be inclined to see mealtime as a task to be accomplished as quickly (but not necessarily as safely) as possible; may delay trays and feeding times until all other residents have been cared for.[5]
Patient is very near death, although may continue to live for months in this condition.	Caregivers may avoid interactions with patient's family because "there is nothing new to report"; fear of "saying the wrong thing"; inability to communicate empathy or consolation.

Here are some questions to ask yourself when searching for ways to cope with the crying out or moaning of late-stage dementia patients. Often, a combination of the following is needed:

a. Could certain areas be especially prepared for patients who cry out, e.g., carpeting on the floor and walls, heavier curtains, and shades?

b. Could these patients be placed closer to the hub of activity where they would receive more attention? Could they be placed farther away from the hub without isolating them from vital caregiving time and attention?

c. Could sound buffers be used to protect other residents from the noise, e.g., sound-proof dividers; assistive listening devices, such as earphones, to focus hearing and attention of other patients?

d. Are there staff members or volunteers who are better at quieting patients in distress? Could more of their time be allocated to these severely demented patients?

e. Is there a time pattern to the patient's crying behavior? Is it possible to plan for these times? Could staff members be available or resources rearranged for these specific times?[4]

f. What types of sensory input do you *consistently* use (not just once or twice) with patients who cry out, i.e., lotions; tape recordings of church or temple music; specific massage techniques (healing touch or myofascial release); hand-holding; stroking; and speaking softly? Some nursing homes are investing in multimedia environmental systems that soothe patients with a combination of soft lighting, specially-recorded music, pleasant aromas, and warm temperatures.

g. Would it make a difference if you consistently tended to these patients' needs—water, food, clean protective garments, and oral hygiene—sooner rather than later?

h. Have you tried light therapy (for persons with certain depressive disorders), better positioning or frequent repositioning (for the immobile), or behavior modification (rewarding the vocalizer for being quiet rather than for being noisy)?[4]

Caregivers have an ethical as well as a professional mandate to continue their efforts to respond to the communication needs of late-stage Alzheimer's disease patients. In spite of their poor response patterns, you must try to communicate with these patients until the end (Recommendation 10.5).

Quick Tip Summary: Difficult Communication Situations
Nonverbal and verbal communication skills are critical in reducing catastrophic reactions of Alzheimer's disease patients. A skillful communication style will also help you deal more effectively with five chronic and irritating behaviors exhibited by Alzheimer's disease patients.

a. Increase your use of nonverbal communication: touch, gesture, and tone of voice.

b. Continue to use adult language and social courtesies when working with and around these patients.

c. Be especially alert for ways to modify the environment (see Units 4 and 5 for more ideas concerning environmental impacts on communication).

d. Increase your reliance on soothing stimuli: music, peaceful videos, lotions, quiet companionship, gentle massage, tape recordings of family voices, parts of church or temple services, laughter, humming, or best loved poems. Explore the possibility of installing a multimedia chamber in your facility.

e. Find a volunteer companion or recorded material that uses the same native language as that of the patient. In the person's last months of life, the sound of one's childhood language may prove to be especially quieting and reassuring.

f. Stay in close communication with family members. They need more assurance than ever that their loved one is being cared for in a proper and caring manner right up to the moment of death.

RECOMMENDATION 10.5   Recommendations for Enhancing Your Communication with Severely Demented Patients

1. *Hallucinations*: Turn hallucinatory incidents into short conversations whenever possible, if the patient is doing no harm to himself or herself or to others.

2. *Repetitive requests or statements*: Select your response based on whether the patient is coping with memory problems or looking for attention. Devise simple memory aids or plan regular personal communication times with the patient.

3. *Resistance or refusal*: Develop communication techniques that enjoin rather than coerce the patient to action. Like most of us, Alzheimer's disease patients resent being directed and controlled.

4. *Wandering and pilfering*: Take a hard look at how well the facility's environment supports patients in finding their way about and whether creative approaches could offer new solutions to wandering and pilfering. Remember, the way a behavior is labeled affects the way it is managed.

5. *Paranoia*: Restore order and reassure everyone involved that their rights and safety are being protected. Your primary communication responsibility is as mediator.

6. *Severe dementia*: Try rearranging the facility's layout, reallocating staff and resources, and exploring different types of calming sensory input. Offer much supportive communication to the family.

REFERENCES

1. Pillemer K, Bachman-Prehn R. Helping and hurting: predictors of maltreatment of patients in nursing homes. Res Aging 1991;13:74.
2. Bourgeois MS. Evaluating memory wallets in conversations with persons with dementia. J Speech Hear Res 1992;35:1344.
3. Smith C, Ventis D. Cooperative and Supportive Behavior of Female Alzheimer's Patients. Paper presented at the annual meeting of the Gerontological Society of America, Boston, 1990.
4. Sloane PD. Managing the patient with disruptive vocalization. Presentation at the Fifth National Alzheimer's Disease Education Conference, Chicago, July 17, 1996.
5. Rajecki, R. Nutritious and fulfilling. Improving residents' eating habits benefits all. Contemp Long Term Care 1993;(Oct):56.

GOOD PRACTICE 10.1   DIFFICULT COMMUNICATION SITUATIONS: WHAT WOULD YOU DO?

Directions: What could you do to improve the communication situation of the individuals described here? Is there anything about the patient's health, environment, emotional, or psychological/social status that could be adjusted so that he or she could be more receptive to your communication?

Grace is in the later stages of Alzheimer's disease. She spends much of the day crying out to anyone passing by. She sees poorly. Although the staff dresses her in clean clothes daily, she often has bits of food in her fingernails, in her hair, and tucked in the crevices of her few remaining teeth. The staff, tired of hearing Grace's shrill voice, wheel her into her room where she bothers fewer people. Suggestions:_____

_____

_____

_____

Paul was admitted to the nursing home shortly after his wife died of cancer. In the middle stages of Alzheimer's disease, he wanders restlessly from room to room asking about Doris. "Have you seen Doris? Do you know where she is?" Some of the other residents become very angry or agitated by his intrusions. Paul seems oblivious to the commotion he sometimes causes. In what way could communication play an important role in managing Paul's behavior? Suggestions:_____

_____

_____

_____

Mabel is mute, although sometimes when her eyes are open, she watches others move about the room. She is kept clean and comfortable but because she causes little trouble, no one spends much time with her. Occasionally, someone gives her a teddy bear to hold. She has no visitors and has lived in the nursing home for 5 years. Why and how should communication still be a part of her life? Suggestions:_____

_____

_____

_____

Antonio moved to the United States when he was 12 years old. He speaks excellent English and was a research scientist in a nearby university. As his disease has progressed, Tony has reverted more and more to his native Italian. He has also become strongly resistant, refusing to dress, to be led to the toilet, to eat with other residents, to do anything cooperatively. He is not combative—yet. There is a church nearby whose pastor is Italian, but Tony's intake sheet declares that he has "no religion."

Suggestions:_____

_____

_____

_____

Bridget frequently accuses staff of stealing or hiding her possessions. She has recently begun to accuse one of the nursing assistants in particular. The young lady is from Manila and possesses excellent caregiving skills and great national pride. She thinks that Bridget is guilty of ethnic slurs. How could this aide use communication to preserve her pride and her job and at the same time appropriately manage Bridget's paranoia?

Suggestions:_____

_____

_____

_____

Positive Techniques for Communicating with Families of Alzheimer's Disease Patients

---

UNIT OUTLINE

Premise

1. Many professional caregivers report that their interactions with patients' families are unpleasant or uncomfortable.
2. Many family members are suspicious or have angry feelings about nursing homes and nursing home employees.
3. Professional caregivers and family members must deal with these feelings if Alzheimer's disease patients are to receive the best treatment.

Definitions

Family Caregiver
Caregiver Burden
Empathetic Listening

**Problems That Family Members Bring to Encounters
with Nursing Home Staff**

1. Negative perception of nursing homes
2. Personal communication problems
3. Long-standing interpersonal communication problems with the patient
4. Confusion over new role
5. Emotional and spiritual neediness

Quick Tip Summary: Communication Problems That Family Caregivers Bring to the Nursing Home

**Problems That Nursing Home Staff Members Bring to
Encounters with Family Members**

Quick Tip Summary: Communication Problems of Staff Members That Cause Family Caregivers to Complain

**Solutions to Conflicts and Positive Techniques for Communicating
with Families of Alzheimer's Disease Patients**

References
Good Practice 11.1 Attitudes and Concerns of Family Members and Professional Caregivers
Good Practice 11.2 Role Play: Interactions with Family Members
Good Practice 11.3 Attending a Support Group Meeting

PREMISE

Many professional caregivers report that their interactions with the families of patients are among the most difficult of their daily duties. In a study of nursing assistants, Richter and his colleagues found many nursing assistants thought that "communicating with the family was the greatest barrier in care of the person with Alzheimer's disease."[1] Nursing assistants commented that families frequently disrupted patient care and were very "demanding." Nursing assistants made statements such as, "It's hard to be nice to the families"; "Family members complain and yell"; "Relatives want attention"; and "Families discuss their feelings of guilt, and I don't know what to say to them."[1]

Clearly, rather than viewing the family as a resource, many of the nursing assistants in Richter's study perceived them to be a major source of stress. At the same time, many family members view nursing homes and nursing home staff with feelings ranging from ambivalence to suspicion, anger, or even contempt. Founded or unfounded, these feelings between professional caregivers and family members must be dealt with if Alzheimer's disease patients are to be provided with the best treatment and if you want to reduce your stress in caregiving.

This unit addresses the question "Why is it so difficult to communicate with patients' families?" by exploring the problems that families bring to the nursing home along with their relatives who have Alzheimer's disease. We will also examine the barriers that staff members bring to encounters with families.

DEFINITIONS

Family Caregiver

The primary family caregiver discussed in this unit is the person in the patient's family who takes primary responsibility for the patient's affairs. Most often this is a female relative, usually the "dutiful daughter." Frequently, this is the person who was providing direct care before the patient entered the nursing home. Fully one-third of primary family caregivers are elderly themselves.

Caregiver Burden

Caregiver burden results from the many physical, psychological, and financial stresses that Alzheimer's disease places on family caregivers. The degree of the burden experienced depends on many interacting factors, but all family caregivers carry a burden.

Empathetic Listening

"Empathetic listening is a nonjudgmental response that captures the essential theme and/or feelings expressed [by the speaker]."[2] Empathetic listening offers the potential for building rapport and mutual understanding between speaker and listener. It does not necessarily indicate agreement or sympathy with the speaker. An example of listening to a family member with empathy might be: "It sounds as though you feel the staff is taking advantage of your willingness to help."

PROBLEMS THAT FAMILY MEMBERS BRING TO ENCOUNTERS WITH NURSING HOME STAFF

1. *Negative perception of nursing homes.* According to one study, at least three-fourths of family caregivers of frail, elderly persons believe that "people go to a nursing home only when there is no other place to live."[3] Family members seem to be unaware of any benefits that a nursing home might provide. Eighty percent of caregivers 70 years old or older see a nursing home as the place of last resort. The less educated, those in poorer health, and those with lower incomes are the most resistant to nursing home placement.

2. *Personal communication problems.* The average age of family caregivers of Alzheimer's disease patients is 57 years. One-third are older than 65. More than two-thirds are women.[4] Elderly family caregivers themselves are at risk for all of the personal communication problems that accompany aging. (See Units 3 and 6.) Many of them are coping with their own hearing losses, depression, aphasia, Parkinson's disease, or other afflictions.

3. *Long-standing interpersonal communication problems with the patient.* By the time a patient enters the nursing home, family members have already experienced profound communication breakdowns, such as the following with the patient. These changes in communication are not as likely to bother the nursing home staff in the same way.

    a. Loss of reciprocity in the relationship; loss of mutual give and take. One daughter reported, "I am stunned by the realization that I'm still playing the role of the criticized child, but she's not playing 'mommy' any more."[5]

b. Asynchronies. When the patient's cycles of sleeping and eating become disturbed, any of the family caregiver's social relationships that centered on mealtimes and bedtimes grind to a halt. For most people, these are the times that in the past had nourished that relationship.

c. Deterioration of social life. As the patient worsens, family caregivers begin to function within a more narrowly constricted social environment. For most family caregivers, this restricted social life does not expand when the patient enters the nursing home.

d. Emotional scars from previous violence. By the time the patient enters the nursing home, communication between family caregiver and patient may have deteriorated so severely that domestic violence has occurred. Research studies have documented patient-to-caregiver physical abuse in 16–33% of cases and caregiver-to-patient violence in 5–23% of cases. The scars of physical abuse are not erased by institutionalization.[6]

4. *Confusion over new role.* Once the patient has been admitted to the nursing home, the role of the family in the patient's care changes radically. In the transition, the family member's status changes from primary caregiver to visitor, from insider to outsider, and from high control to low control over the patient's care. At the same time, the majority of family members continue to have frequent contact with their loved ones after admission and perceive that their burden of care continues after institutionalization. In truth, "the family is often working through feelings of loss, guilt, and helplessness and may have a strong need to continue the caregiving role after a loved one has been admitted to the nursing home."[1]

Many family members view themselves as protectors or advocates for their loved ones in the nursing home and want to provide as much of the hands-on care as possible. However, families are not usually oriented to the procedures of a long-term care facility and learn only by trial and error what duties they may and may not assume. If a nursing home does not provide clear guidelines for families regarding their roles and responsibilities, ambiguity and conflict are likely to occur. Some family members think that too many patient care duties are still left to them despite the fact that they are paying a large amount of money to the nursing home. According to Maas et al.,[7] family members react to ambiguous situations with hostility toward staff, disagreements over the use of services, criticism of the care provided, and less frequent visits. They also react with increased guilt, health problems, and more use of drugs and medications.

5. *Emotional and spiritual neediness.* Families of Alzheimer's disease patients must make many emotional and spiritual adjustments during the course of the disease. The most common are:

a. The need to deal with their own feelings of guilt and sadness at having institutionalized the patient. Many Alzheimer's disease patients remain at home far beyond the point at which admission to the nursing home might have been optimal and far beyond the breaking point for family caregivers. Usually, there is dissension in the family over the placement, and often the person who makes the final decision is berated by the patient and by the rest of the family. The feelings of guilt, anger, and mourning that this process engenders do not suddenly evaporate after the admission. They reappear in the family caregiver's search for reassurance, denial of earlier problems, and defensiveness in interacting with professional caregiving staff.

b. The search for remaining connectedness to the patient. Because it is so difficult to deal with the loss of communication with a mate, a parent, or a sibling, most family members continue to work hard to stay connected with the patient. They will state with conviction, "I'm sure he knew it was me sitting with him even though he couldn't say my name." Connectedness is extremely important to them.

c. The search for meaning in the disease. By the time an Alzheimer's disease patient enters the nursing home, family members have spent a great deal of effort trying to find some meaning in their loved one's illness. After they have turned over their caregiving role to the institution, this search for meaning may become all-consuming.

d. The need to grieve over the slow loss of a loved one and to deal with his or her ultimate death. Under any circumstances, death is the most difficult event that humans face. Psychologists tell us that most people find it more difficult to deal with the deaths of their loved ones than with their own deaths. Family caregivers of Alzheimer's disease patients have already begun to deal with this reality. Their loved ones are slipping away day by day, yet many nursing homes barely acknowledge the pain of death and the need to grieve. Many do not even offer a memorial service when a patient dies. This silence discredits the importance of the family's loved one and the enormity of the family's feelings of grief.

e. The need to grieve over personal losses of health, quality of life, financial resources, and affection that occur over the course of long-term caregiving. Perhaps the most poignant adjustment of all for caregivers is to the reality that, even though responsibility for the loved one has been delegated to a nursing home, the personal toll for years of caregiving has been life-changing and, in some ways, permanent. The primary caregiver has had to constantly redefine his or her life in the knowledge that the partner can no longer accept or confer affection and moral support. The illness endlessly soaks up vital savings and investments and arbitrarily turns simple pleasures and social routines into nightmare performances. Inevitably, the primary caregiver's quality of life and health status suffer. Once the patient is relocated or gone forever, that family member has to confront those personal losses and grieve for them.

Quick Tip Summary: Communication Problems That Family Caregivers Bring to the Nursing Home

1. Negative perceptions of nursing homes; at least three-fourths of Americans see nursing homes as a last resort.
2. Personal communication problems of the family caregiver; caregivers also suffer from hearing loss, depression, Parkinson's disease, and other problems associated with aging.
3. Additional long-standing communication problems with the Alzheimer's disease patient, such as:
   a. Loss of reciprocity.
   b. "Asynchronies"—loss of mealtime and bedtime relationships.
   c. Deterioration of social life.
   d. Emotional scars from previous domestic violence.
4. Confusion over the transition in role from primary caregiver to visitor.
5. Spiritual and emotional neediness, which includes:
   a. Need to deal with their own feelings of guilt and sadness at having institutionalized the patient.
   b. Need to remain "connected" to the patient.
   c. Need to find meaning in the disease.
   d. Need to grieve over the slow loss of a loved one.
   e. Need to grieve over personal losses of health, quality of life, financial resources, and affection.

PROBLEMS THAT NURSING HOME STAFF MEMBERS BRING TO ENCOUNTERS WITH FAMILY MEMBERS

What is it that members of the nursing home staff do, or do not do, that causes communication to break down with family members? Family members who participated in the Maas et al. study[7] reported that what caused them the most dissatisfaction with the nursing home was the failure of staff members to solicit their help with care. They were also distressed when staff members were too busy to give needed care or too busy to make sure that their loved one was involved in patient activities.

Family caregivers also complained that staff caregivers viewed the job of caregiving as simply doing tasks for the patients; that they worked only to maintain the institutional routine and control, having little consideration for the needs of the patient. Families thought that staff members "type-cast" them, avoided them, and disregarded their importance to the patient.

Whether all of this is true is less important than whether family members *believe* it is true. Family caregivers act on their beliefs; and family members' beliefs about the care of their relatives are based almost entirely on the quality of their own interactions with staff caregivers. They appear to assess quality of care by how well the staff protects the dignity and individuality of the patient.[8]

There are also some unpleasant realities in how staff members in many nursing homes interact with families. Most staff members are not well equipped to deal with the problems that families bring to the nursing home. Direct care staff often have little preparation for dealing with grieving families and little knowledge of the family history of each patient. They have a hard enough time getting to know each patient.

Quick Tip Summary: Communication Problems of Staff Members That Cause Family Caregivers to Complain

1. Staff members fail to ask family members for help with the care of the patient.
2. Staff members appear too busy to provide adequate care.
3. Staff members do not know patients well and do not get them to appropriate activities.
4. Staff members work for the institution and not for the family. They ignore the family's needs.
5. Staff members "dump" too many patient care duties on them.
6. Staff members "type-cast" families, avoid them, or disregard their importance to the patient.

SOLUTIONS TO CONFLICTS AND POSITIVE TECHNIQUES FOR COMMUNICATING WITH FAMILIES OF ALZHEIMER'S DISEASE PATIENTS

To reduce conflicts, both staff and family members have to make adjustments. Two things must happen: first, staff members must become sensitive to the family's anxiety; second, family members must be willing to relinquish the primary caregiver role.

One of the best ways for direct care staff members to pay attention to the family's concerns and to ease tension is to practice empathetic listening skills. As defined earlier in this unit, empathetic listening seeks to capture or validate the feelings of the speaker and to build rapport rather than to defend or argue a particular point. Empathetic listening responses are usually effective in easing the level of emotional tension and helpful in allowing individuals to clarify their positions (Recommendation 11.1). Empathetic responses also encourage family members to solve their own problems. The following phrases will help you shape your own empathetic responses with family members:

- "It sounds as if you're—"
- "You seem to be—"
- "What I'm hearing from you is—"
- "I sense that—"
- "You must have felt—"
- "Let me see if I understand—"
- "That does present a problem."

Before relatives can relinquish their primary caregiver status, they need reassurance that their loved ones are being cared for as well as, or better than, at home. You, the professional caregiver, must assume responsibility for communicating that reassurance (Recommendation 11.2).

a. Convey a positive attitude through your nonverbal behavior: maintain eye contact; assume an interested facial expression; and use open, non-threatening body postures and gestures, such as head nods and light touch. Avoid body language that inadvertently intimidates: don't turn your back, cross your arms, frown, sigh, or roll your eyes. Reinforce your nonverbal behavior with encouraging verbal responses, such as "Oh," "Yes, I see," or "Um-hmm."

b. Ask as few direct questions as possible. You do not want the person to have the feeling of being interrogated or that you are not going to believe any statement unless you have heard the last shred of evidence. You may be surprised to learn that your empathetic listening responses and open body language are just as effective as direct questions for finding out what you need to know.

c. Use open-ended requests to show your interest. For instance:
"Can you give me an example?"
"Let's talk about this in private."
"Please tell me more."
"I'd like to hear what you have to say. Come back at about 2:00, when I can spend more time with you."
"I always value your opinion (observations)."

d. See if the complaining family caregiver can become part of the solution instead of one who only defines the problem. Try requests such as:
"What have you already tried?"
"Tell me some of your ideas for working this out."
"Do you know other people who would be willing to help with this?"
"Would you like to bring your questions (concerns) directly to (the doctor, floor nurse, administrator)? I'd be happy to help (or to find someone else to help)."

e. Avoid:
   i. Jumping in with a quick solution or advice before you understand what the "real problem" is. The family member may be talking about one issue but actually be angry about another.
   ii. Interrupting.
   iii. Trying to distract the person with unrelated information.
   iv. Using stereotyped "Band-Aid" statements, e.g., "I know just how you feel." "Isn't that just like a man (woman)?" "That's just the way it is. I can't change it." "Well, we all have our troubles." "Must be a full moon."
   v. Becoming defensive, e.g., "You have no idea how hard our job is in this facility." "You can't talk to me that way." "It was just a little push in the right direction. Anyway, he hit me first."
   vi. Criticizing or belittling the family member's feelings or the complaint, e.g., "You shouldn't let yourself get so upset." "I can't understand why this is bothering you." "Well, this isn't the first time (patient's name) has done that."
   vii. Spreading toxic talk (see Unit 8 for a definition) around the facility about relatives who are "troublemakers," "always complaining," or "impossible to deal with."

RECOMMENDATION 11.1   Recommendations for Empathetic Listening

a. See the patient as a member of a family unit. View the family as an extension of the patient. Keep the family informed about the patient's likes, dislikes, and adjustment to life in the nursing home.

b. Engage the family's participation in the patient's care from the beginning. Families can be a good source of information. For example, a family member can tell you much about a patient's eating habits—what foods he or she likes and dislikes, whether the big family meal is at midday or at night, whether the patient likes to snack, whether the patient prefers hot or cold food. Sometimes family members can help feed the patient. A husband or wife may take great pride in how well he or she is able to get the spouse to eat (Illustration 11.1).

c. Provide support for the family during the difficult period of role transition. There are many ways to support families during transition.

    i. Be willing to listen to families during the period of adjustment. You do not have to stop what you are doing, just let them know you are listening while you work. Usually families do not expect you to give them advice; they just need to talk. Since most primary family caregivers have a restricted social life, you might be the only person available who understands their situation.

    ii. Help them "learn the ropes" of the nursing home; empower them whenever possible. Families need to know, for example, to whom they should go with a complaint. Sometimes families take small complaints, such as lost laundry, toileting, or mistakes in the patient's diet, noisily to the administrator of the nursing home because they do not know who is directly responsible.

    iii. Make suggestions for things to do during family visits. Having observed successful visitors over time, you can suggest to family members activities such as brushing or grooming their relative's hair, watching a home video together, praying or singing, and so on.

    iv. Encourage families to attend support groups. Good support groups can reduce family members' isolation and help them realize that their relative is being cared for as well as or better than he or she would be at home.

    v. Visit a family support group meeting to better understand the self-help process.

RECOMMENDATION 11.2   Recommendations for Reassuring Family Members That Their Relative Is Receiving Good Care

Exasperated, the head nurse stands eye-to-eye with Morris, who sits confused on the side of his new nursing home bed. Holding a paper cup in one hand and two pills in the other, she looks helplessly over his shoulder as his wife, Shirley, enters the sun-filled room.

"We've tried everything," the nurse laments to the wife. "We cannot get him to take his medication. I don't know what we're going to do. How did you ever manage him at home?" "I didn't have a problem with that," Shirley responds calmly. She takes the cup and pills from the nurse and places them in her husband's two hands. She walks over to the sink and gets a paper cup of water for herself. Smiling, she caresses the side of Morris' face until he is looking directly at her. She lifts her cup in the air for a toast, shouts "Cheers!" pretends to put pills in her mouth, then drinks down the water.

"Cheers!" Morris declares, raising his cup. Down go the pills; down goes the water. He hands Shirley the cup with a satisfied smile and lies back down on the bed, untroubled. (Reprinted with permission from MJ Santo Pietro. Assessing the communicative styles of caregivers of patients with Alzheimer's disease. Semin Speech Lang 1994;15;236.)

Illustration 11.1   Family Participation in Patient Care

REFERENCES

1. Richter J, Bottenberg D, Roberto K. Communication between formal caregivers and individuals with Alzheimer's disease. Am J Alzheimer's Care Rel Dis Res 1993;8:25.
2. Burley-Allen M. Listening, The Forgotten Skill. New York: Wiley, 1982;89.
3. Cafferata G, Stone R. Community caregivers' attitudes toward nursing homes. J Long-Term Care Admin 1991–1992;(Winter):33.
4. Rau M. Impact on Families. In R Lubinski (ed), Dementia and Communication. Philadelphia: BC Decker, 1991;153.
5. Lynch-Sauer J. When a family member has Alzheimer's disease: a phenomenological description of caregiving. J Gerontol Nurs 1989;16:9.
6. Paneza GJ, Cohan D, Eisdorfer C. Severe family violence and Alzheimer's disease: Prevalence and risk factors. Gerontologist 32;4:493.
7. Maas M, Buckwalter D, Kelley J, Stolley J. Family members' perceptions: how they view care of Alzheimer's patients in a nursing home. J Long-term Care Admin 1991;(Spring);21.
8. Johnson M. Daughter's responses to a parent's relocation to a nursing home. Paper presented at the 42nd Annual Scientific Meeting of the Gerontological Society of America. Minneapolis, 1989.

PRACTICE 11.1   ATTITUDES AND CONCERNS OF FAMILY MEMBERS AND PROFESSIONAL CAREGIVERS

Directions: Indicate whether the following statements best describe family caregivers (FC), nursing home staff caregivers (SC), or both (B). What do your answers tell you about the differences or similarities between family and professional caregivers?

___ 1. Most believe that nursing homes are places for old people who have no other place to live.

___ 2. They are frequently overwhelmed by the responsibilities and stresses of the daily duties of caregiving.

___ 3. They continue to feel responsible for the patient when they are no longer primary caregivers.

___ 4. They tend to judge the quality of the patient's care by the way in which the caregiver interacts with and protects the dignity and individuality of the patient.

___ 5. They generally have inadequate preparation for dealing with the communication problems of the Alzheimer's disease patient and of other caregivers.

___ 6. If they feel they are not in control of the patient, they criticize the other caregivers.

___ 7. They are sometimes reluctant to share knowledge about the patient's personal life and preferences with other caregivers.

___ 8. They may know best how to communicate appropriately with the Alzheimer's disease patient.

___ 9. Their efforts to spend time conversing with the Alzheimer's disease patient are important to the patient's well-being.

___ 10. When a resident dies, memorial services at the nursing home might assist them in the grieving process.

GOOD PRACTICE 11.2   ROLE PLAY: INTERACTIONS WITH FAMILY MEMBERS

Directions: Select two or three of the following role-play scenarios and have the group read and discuss the communication problems they might encounter in each situation. Then select students to play the roles. If the group is familiar with role-playing activities, the roles of a family member and a staff person can be played by individuals in the group. If role playing is a new experience for the group, the instructor should take the part of the family member.

Note to instructors: Refer to detailed guidelines for facilitating effective role-playing exercises in "Introduction to Instructors" at the beginning of this manual.

1. *Keep the family informed about the patient's adjustment to the nursing home environment.* Since being placed in the nursing home, Harry has been extremely resistant and restless; a month has gone by and he still has not settled into a routine. The staff has tried several things to ease his behavior, but you suspect that Harry is also feeling displaced and isolated. His son and other family members rarely visit, and then only for brief moments. You want to enlist his son's help in finding solutions. Now you see him hurriedly entering Harry's room. How are you going to approach him? Given his constant rush, how much will you be able to say?

2. *Engage family participation in patient care from the beginning.* Peggy is willing to take time off from work 5 days a week to feed her mother at lunch. You are grateful until you see what her feeding skills are like. She feeds rapidly, puts too much food on the spoon, distracts her mother constantly instead of helping her to focus on safe chewing, swallowing, and meal completion, even occasionally gives her bites that are too hot. Her mother is often in a state of acute distress by the end of a meal.

Your options are to tell Peggy that she is no longer welcome to feed her mother, to refer her to your supervisor, or to offer some gentle instruction and demonstration of how to feed her mother safely and pleasantly. How can you employ one of these options without offending Peggy in her role of family caregiver?

3. *Provide support for the family during role transition; be willing to listen to family members during the period of adjustment.* Mrs. Collister is wonderfully supportive of the staff but feels guilty about placing her husband in the home. She attends the nursing home support meetings but also wants to interact with the nursing assistants who care directly for her husband. What active listening techniques, as one of the nursing assistants, can you use to comfort her as she speaks of her worries?

4. *Help family members learn the ropes. Let them know how they can help, and to whom they can complain.* Mr. Robbins' daughter, Janice, is complaining loudly about how his television has been moved again, after she has repeatedly moved it to a spot in the room where he can see it best. You are the person who has been returning the set to its original spot on the basis of safety regulations, which state that electrical wires cannot extend over a certain number of feet from their source. You suspect that her anger actually stems from no longer having control over her father's life and environment.

Are you going to handle this interaction merely as a safety issue? If you are not the best person to handle her complaint, how can you guide her? Can you offer some solutions that would not interfere with your routine but would give her some sense of control?

5. *Make suggestions for things to do during family visits.* Mrs. Ames' two nieces are young, cheery, and a good antidote for their very confused aunt. Tell the girls about two or three activities that their aunt might enjoy attending. Describe the activities in a way that shows how the nieces could be of real help, e.g., transporting her to activities, staying with her so she will not wander, keeping her hands busy so that she does not pick, and reading to her at a time when she tends to nag the staff. How can you guide them to more productive use of the time with their aunt?

6. *Encourage family members to attend family support groups.* Mr. Jones took care of his wife for years before finally placing her in the nursing home but has never joined a support group. When he visits Mrs. Jones, which is frequently, he expects busy staff members to listen while he talks endlessly about his wife and every caregiving mistake or victory he ever had. You are a good listener and are happy to have some of the information, but his lengthy monologues are beginning to intrude on your tight schedule.

You recently attended a meeting of the nursing home's support group and were impressed by the participants' sharing of information. How would you encourage Mr. Jones to try it, too?

GOOD PRACTICE 11.3   ATTENDING A SUPPORT GROUP MEETING

Directions: Attend one or two meetings of your nursing home's support group for family members of patients with Alzheimer's disease. Go with one of your coworkers if possible. Together, answer the following questions and report your insights to your supervisor at the next staff meeting or at the next in-service training session on communication skills.

1. What was the location like where the meeting was held? Was there a comfortable atmosphere, e.g., good lighting, comfortable seating, and good acoustics? Was the place distraction-free, e.g., no calling system, television noise, or traffic through the room?_____

_____

_____

_____

2. Did you let the group know ahead of time that you were going to attend? Did you feel like an "outsider" or did you feel comfortably included? Were you personally introduced? Was there a general introduction when everyone said who they were or why they were attending or did this seem to be a "set" group where people took it for granted that "everyone knows everyone else"?_____

_____

_____

_____

3. Was the group facilitator a lay person, a professional health-care worker from outside your nursing home, or an employee of your facility? Did he or she encourage people to "vent," "complain," and "commiserate" about the burdens of caregiving, or did the facilitator guide people toward finding and sharing solutions to their problems?_____

_____

_____

4. What observations did you make about the communication styles of certain group members? Refer to earlier sections of this unit and Unit 5 for assistance in answering this question. Did anyone seem to have a communication disorder—hearing loss, dysarthria, Parkinson's disease—that caused speech problems? Did anyone have a communication style that was especially difficult for you to under-

stand—foreign accent, rapid speech, mumbling, or overuse of complicated words?_____

_____

_____

_____

5. Was there a speaker? (Is there usually a speaker?) If so, what was the speaker's topic? How favorably was the information received by the other guests? As a caregiver, did you find the information useful or interesting?_____

_____

_____

6. What do you think was the most valuable aspect of this support group meeting? Having attended a meeting, how do you now feel about recommending the support group to your patients' families? What changes or improvements would you make if you were in charge?_____

_____

_____

UNIT 12

Direct Intervention Programs for Alzheimer's Disease Patients: Increasing Their Communication Opportunities in the Nursing Home

UNIT OUTLINE

Premise

1. Good clinical practice is always based on sound research principles.
2. If patients with Alzheimer's disease have few or no opportunities to use retained communication skills, their relative communication strengths begin to diminish from disuse.
3. There are several research-tested programs that intervene directly with caregivers or patients for the purpose of maximizing patients' communication skills.

Definitions

Communication Opportunity

Direct Communication Intervention Programs

Providing Communication Opportunities: What Is Communication Intervention and Why Should We Provide It?

Communication Interventions That Have Proved Effective in Nursing Home Settings

1. Memory Books or wallets
2. Conversation groups
3. The Breakfast Club
4. Communication Partners
5. The FOCUSED Program for Caregivers

Developing Intervention Techniques for Effective Communication with Alzheimer's Patients in All Situations

References

Good Practice 12.1 Implementing a Direct Intervention Program: Group Discussion

PREMISE

Good clinical practice is always based on sound research principles. It is well known that Alzheimer's disease patients respond best when they reside in a safe and predictable physical environment and are cared for by calm, supportive personnel. This management philosophy has been discovered through clinical experience and through the rigorous research of health care investigators.[1]

Communication skills are like most other human abilities—you must "use them or lose them." For persons with Alzheimer's disease, the adage should read "use them or lose them faster." If patients with Alzheimer's disease have few or no opportunities to use retained communication skills, the relative strengths described in Unit 2 (procedural memories, social rituals, etc.) diminish at a quicker rate from disuse. Instead of learning to maintain function with the skills remaining, patients learn helplessness. In fact, family members and professional caregivers often directly contribute to learned helplessness. (See Unit 2 for a definition of learned helplessness.) Out of genuine concern for the patient's safety and well-being, caregivers prevent patients from engaging in activities that would allow them to exercise their remaining skills.

This unit acquaints you with a number of research-tested methods for offering Alzheimer's disease patients opportunities for maintaining their communication skills. All have been tested and used in the nursing home setting.

DEFINITIONS

Communication Opportunity
A communication opportunity is any encounter that offers the possibility for "good communication" between two persons. A communication opportunity might be a passing moment of contact in the hallway, a Sunday afternoon visit, or a planned group social activity.

Direct Communication Intervention Program
Direct communication intervention programs are specific, defined approaches that provide encouraging communication opportunities for persons with Alzheimer's disease.

PROVIDING COMMUNICATION OPPORTUNITIES: WHAT IS COMMUNICATION INTERVENTION AND WHY SHOULD WE PROVIDE IT?

Increased attention is being paid to direct intervention programs that help patients maintain or even improve their levels of communication. Although research on the topic is new, several treatment techniques appear to be having success. Successful intervention attempts to achieve the following goals:

1. Maintain as many of an Alzheimer's disease patient's residual functional communication strengths as possible.
2. Prevent overreaction to disability or learned helplessness.
3. Relieve the burden of caregiving; maintain the health and integrity of the caregiver.
4. Improve the quality of life for and maintain the human dignity of both patient and caregiver.
5. Establish harmonious functioning within the nursing home setting.

Many caregivers believe there is no point in trying to work with Alzheimer's disease patients through formal intervention programs: "They are only going to get worse." "They don't remember anything you teach them." "They're confused." But Alzheimer's disease patients are living longer and longer, and we are living with them. We need to communicate with them, and they have a great need to communicate with us. Direct intervention programs offer caregivers specific guidelines for trying and then carefully evaluating the results of particular ways to communicate. As long as there are persons with Alzheimer's disease, there will be a need to seek formal and informal methods of improving communication between patient and caregiver.

COMMUNICATION INTERVENTIONS THAT HAVE PROVED EFFECTIVE IN NURSING HOME SETTINGS

Several promising, new communication treatments can be implemented by direct care staff with guidance from communication specialists. Of the five treatment plans discussed here, three target the patient's communication skills and two seek to enhance the caregiver's communication skills.

1. Communication notebooks or wallets[2, 3]
2. Communication partners[4]
3. The conversation group[5]

4. The Breakfast Club[6, 7]
5. The FOCUSED Program for Caregivers[8]

For more detailed information about each treatment, consult the references at the end of this unit.

All five treatment protocols were developed using the guidelines below. In choosing a communication intervention for *patients,* keep the following advice in mind:

1. Choose activities that practice everyday communication skills, ones that recur in the patient's daily life and that the environment will support.
2. Choose activities that match the everyday routines of the nursing home (e.g., do not rely on a single caregiver to provide the activities if there is a large turnover of personnel; do not work on singing if patients are required to keep quiet).
3. Choose activities that capitalize on the patient's remaining abilities.

In choosing a communication intervention for *caregivers,* keep the following advice in mind:

1. Target communication behaviors that are likely to occur in the everyday repertoire of the caregiver and the patient.
2. Target communication behaviors that are achievable and have tangible results.
3. Match the goals of the program to the level of the patient with whom the caregiver is communicating.

Memory Books or Wallets

Many speech-language pathologists working in nursing homes have found that making a "memory notebook" as described by Mateer and Sohlberg[2] or a "memory wallet" as described by Bourgeois[3] is extremely helpful in providing communication opportunities for patients with Alzheimer's disease.

The *memory notebook* involves the assembly of current, pertinent information about the patient and his or her present surroundings: name, room number, schedule, roommate, and family pictures with names. The book also includes references to events and pictures from the past—information about who that person was before he or she became ill. Information is printed in simple, declarative sentences; pictures are captioned with simple, identifying sentences.

The memory notebook serves many purposes. It takes advantage of the patient's ability to read single words. It helps to maintain present orientation as well as early life memories. Caregivers can use the notebook: (1) as a daily review with the patient, (2) as a source of the patient's history, (3) as a tool for informal conversation, or (4) as a means of encouraging interaction between patients. If visitors pause to comment on the book, the patient has additional opportunities to communicate.

The *memory wallet* also includes personal information and photographs but in a more portable form. Bourgeois taught caregivers to train middle-stage Alzheimer's disease patients in the use of memory wallets. Several of her studies were performed with nursing home patients and their professional caregivers. Caregivers asked the patients simple questions that could be answered with information in the wallet. Within 3 months, patients learned that when they could not answer questions, they should reach for their memory wallets. Bourgeois found that even though the deterioration caused by Alzheimer's disease continued, these patients began to use more statements of fact and more "novel utterances," and they sought conversation more frequently after they had their wallets.

Conversation Groups

Conversation groups give Alzheimer's disease patients "a means to establish an interpersonal situation in which meaningful, motivating, and reinforcing communication can occur."[9] Being present in a group serves to stimulate a patient's verbalizations, to increase interactions, and to renew group members as independent participants. Group sessions can take many forms: reminiscence, current events, games, problem solving, or free exchanges of ideas and experiences (Recommendation 12.1).

The Breakfast Club

The Breakfast Club is a group communication intervention that incorporates everything known about effective communication with nursing home patients with Alzheimer's disease. Developed by Boczko,[6] the Breakfast Club is a directed activity in which a small group of Alzheimer's disease patients prepares, serves, and eats breakfast and cleans up afterward. Ideally, the 45-minute meetings are held five mornings a week in a homelike kitchen setting that is carefully controlled for visual and auditory distractions. Five residents who have not yet had breakfast are seated around a rectangular table with the facilitator at one end.

To avoid sensory overload and confusion, the program's food choices are limited and include only those items the participants are capable of preparing. Tasks progress from simple ones (i.e., choosing butter or jam for toast) to more complex ones (i.e., actually making French toast or pancakes and flipping them on the griddle) as the weeks go on.

a. Conversation groups for Alzheimer's disease patients work best when there is one facilitator per four or five participants.

b. Participants should be seated around a table and some food should be served. This physical arrangement helps maintain focus and attention.[5]

c. The table should be in the corner of the room. The walls give patients a feeling of stability and security. Wanderers can be seated in the corner so that leaving is less inviting.

d. A "crier" should be removed from a conversation group if the activity does not have a quieting effect on the person after the second session.

e. Name tags with large print should be provided for each member. Members should be referred to frequently by name.

Additional Recommendations for Group Conversation Intervention with Middle-Stage Alzheimer's Disease Patients

a. Speak slowly, loudly, and clearly.

b. Use stimuli that are tangible and of real interest to the group. Have things (e.g., pictures, objects, or printed words) on the table so that members may look at, touch, and pass them around.

c. Provide rewards and positive feedback. Every member's effort to speak should be supported and reinforced.

d. Do not force or correct responses. The patient's error is at least an attempt to communicate and should be greeted positively.

e. Progress from simple to more complex in all activities. (Example: Pass around a pot of flowers; touch, smell, and name the parts. Then pass and comment on items for planting. Finally, plant some flowers in a new pot.)

f. Encourage group members to do most of the talking, especially to each other. Avoid a classroom "question and answer" format whenever possible.

g. Make new information an extension of the familiar.

h. Develop a theme (i.e., holidays, hearing aids, wedding anniversaries, or child-rearing practices) but allow the patients' responses to dictate the course of the conversation.

i. Summarize and restate points frequently. Help keep the participants on topic.

j. Offer opportunities to each member to join in the group at his or her own level of communication ability.

RECOMMENDATION 12.1 Recommendations for Conducting Conversation Groups with Alzheimer's Disease Patients
(Adapted from L Clark, K Witte. Nature and Efficacy of Communication Management in Alzheimer's Disease. In R Lubinski [ed], Dementia and Communication. Philadelphia: BC Decker, 1991;238.)

The Breakfast Club seeks to provide patients with the following specific benefits: (a) maintenance of organizational, decision-making skills; (b) maintenance of conversational and social skills; (c) maintenance of early life memories; (d) maintenance of interest and involvement; (e) facilitation of retained procedural memories; (f) facilitation of retained language abilities and reading skills; (g) stimulation of hearing, vision, smell, taste, and touch; (h) stimulation of positive emotions; (i) prevention of learned helplessness; and (j) prevention of isolation and premature deterioration of communication skills.

The Breakfast Club follows a structured format from beginning to end with a 10-step protocol that includes greetings, choices of juices and breakfast foods, joint preparation of coffee and breakfast, serving of coffee and breakfast entree, clean up, conversation over coffee, and leave-taking. In the beginning, patients only do as much of the preparation and cleanup as they are able, but greater levels of independence are encouraged over time.

Throughout the Breakfast Club sessions, the group leader uses generous amounts of feedback and positive reinforcement and incorporates language stimulation strategies, such as choice questions and closure. (See Unit 9 for definitions of *choice questions* and *closure*.) The leader's language style encourages, inspires, and animates the patients with words that convey warmth and acceptance, yet the style definitely reflects an adult attitude. The leader does not try to control every interaction. By being a good listener, the leader encourages patients to initiate conversation and to talk to one another as well as to the leader.

Preliminary research results on the effectiveness of the Breakfast Club are impressive. Over a 12-week period, Breakfast Club participants in the Jewish Home and Hospital for Aged in Bronx, New York, not only improved in the use of language and communication skills, but also showed renewed use of procedural memories for preparing, sharing, and eating a meal and significantly more independence and calmness in their everyday lives. Their social ritual abilities resurfaced, and they began to show genuine social concern for one another[10] (Illustration 12.1).

Communication Partners

Communication Partners is a communication intervention program initially developed by Lyon for use with elderly post-stroke patients.[4] In this program a volunteer is trained to communicate more successfully with the communication-impaired patient. For the program to work with an Alzheimer's disease patient, the volunteer should master techniques such as those presented in Units 9 and 10.

Week 1: The nursing staff expressed reservations about Gertrude's participation in the experimental group. She was isolated and uncooperative on the unit. In the early sessions, Gertrude appeared frightened and frustrated and remained silent most of the time. She refused to try to crack her egg. She could not spread jelly on toast even with coaching from the leader.

Week 2: Gertrude became so upset one day at the prospect of participating that she left the room.

Week 3: Gertrude smiled and independently cracked her egg. When the facilitator asked her to help Miriam, she responded, "No. Mine's okay, hers is something else." But at the end of the session, she said to Miriam, "Come on, Miriam, are you ready to go?"

Week 7: Gertrude held the door open for other members and told everyone it was her job. Then she walked in and pointed to her chair and said, "That's my chair." She commented on Jack's cracking of his egg, "He's cracking it right, but it's taking him a long time."

Week 8: When Mildred passed out utensils, Gertrude commented, "That's a girl. You're doing a great job!"

Week 10: Gertrude showed her name tag to everyone and crowed, "This is my name and it's a good one."

Week 12: At a meeting of the nursing staff on the unit, a nursing assistant remarked, "Gertrude is so much more cooperative. She can really follow directions now."

Illustration 12.1   Gertrude and the Breakfast Club

Volunteers are first sought from among the patient's friends. A second source might be the nursing home's volunteer service or the members of a local senior center or church. Fellow residents who are cognitively intact also make excellent and available volunteers. Once the volunteer is comfortable communicating with the patient, a regular program of communication opportunities is planned. Activities might include in-room visits or games, walks, gardening, or trips outside the nursing home. Whenever possible, the activities should cater to the patient's preferences and reinforce the patient's remaining independence and communication skills. Volunteer visits might be once a day or once a week.

Although memory books, conversation groups, and the Breakfast Club are most helpful for patients who are in the middle stages of Alzheimer's disease, a Communication Partners program can serve Alzheimer's disease patients up through their final hours. Sitting with a late-stage patient in quiet companionship, stroking the patient's hair, singing softly or humming, or helping to feed or calm the patient during the last days are wonderfully human ways of extending a Communication Partners project. If a Communication

Partners program is begun early enough in the stay of an Alzheimer's disease patient, the patient could have a familiar companion throughout the entire ordeal of decline.

The FOCUSED Program for Caregivers

The FOCUSED program, developed by Ripich,[8] is a caregiver intervention program that has proven effective in fostering positive communication exchanges between nursing home staff members and patients with Alzheimer's disease. It employs nonverbal and verbal communication strategies and, like the Communication Partners program, can be used throughout the entire course of the disease. Directed to family and professional caregivers, it incorporates seven general communication strategies into a framework that can be recalled and applied by the use of the acronym, FOCUSED: *F*ace the person; *O*rient to the topic; *C*ontinue the topic; *U*nstick communication blocks; *S*tructure with questions; *E*xchange conversation; use *D*irect statements.

Each of these strategies represents a set of techniques that must be mastered to put the program into effect. The techniques can be learned from a caregiver manual developed by Ripich and Wykle and listed in the references at the end of this chapter.[8]

DEVELOPING INTERVENTION TECHNIQUES FOR EFFECTIVE COMMUNICATION WITH ALZHEIMER'S PATIENTS IN ALL SITUATIONS

Once you have a clear understanding of the communication problems and strengths of Alzheimer's disease patients as well as your own communication problems and strengths, you can work to create your own mini-interventions with elderly patients with dementia. Below is a list of 20 general "dos and don'ts" to help you achieve successful communication with your Alzheimer's disease patients.

Dos and Don'ts for Maintaining Successful Communication with Alzheimer's Disease Patients

1. *Use adult language.* You are communicating with adult patients. Patients are apt to respond negatively when you address them as children, no matter how kindly you intend to be. To help the patient maintain self-respect, use an adult communication style .

2. *Maintain eye contact.* Alzheimer's disease patients need as many nonverbal cues as possible. Eye contact is vital for maximum communication. If the patient is not looking at you, establish eye contact by calling his or her name or gently touching the patient's arm. Always stand face-to-face with an Alzheimer's disease patient

when speaking. If the patient is in a wheelchair, bring yourself down to the patient at eye level.

3. *Use visual cues whenever possible.* There is evidence to show that Alzheimer's disease patients continue to respond appropriately to visual communication longer than spoken communication. Written words, pictures, gestures, and facial expressions all help to get information across to patients with Alzheimer's disease.

4. *Use simple words and short sentences.* Simple words remain available to Alzheimer's disease patients longer than difficult ones, and short sentences are easier to comprehend than complex ones.

5. *Keep your explanations short.* Alzheimer's disease patients are more likely to complete some longer tasks if the tasks are broken into single-step directions. For example: "Pick up the spoon. Put the spoon in the bowl."

6. *Paraphrase, do not just repeat.* If the patient has difficulty understanding a message, find a different way to say it rather than repeating the original words over and over. Other words might be more meaningful.

7. *Avoid saying, "Don't you remember?"* Chances are, the patient does not. Constant reminders that the patient's memory is failing can be very distressing for both patient and caregiver.

8. *Use touch.* Guidance, reassurance, affection, and humor can be communicated to an Alzheimer's disease patient through touch even in the later stages of the disease.

9. *Do not shout.* If hearing is not a problem, your tone of voice may frighten the patient or put the patient in a defensive mood. If hearing is a problem, shouting distorts your message. Many hearing-impaired elderly patients also suffer from *tinnitus* (ringing in the ears) or *recruitment* (an inability to hear soft noises while loud noises are perceived at their actual level of loudness). Shouting at persons with tinnitus or recruitment makes the problems worse and stresses the patient.

10. *Do not interrupt.* Try not to interrupt unless it is absolutely necessary. If you interrupt an Alzheimer's disease patient in the middle of an attempt to communicate or in the middle of a task, it is likely that the patient will forget what he or she was saying or doing. Alzheimer's disease patients are easily distracted, even when they are speaking or acting with firm intent.

11. *Avoid competition.* Avoid competing signals, such as television, radio, or other conversations. If you have something really important to tell an Alzheimer's disease patient, speak to the person face-to-face in a quiet place.

12. *Use a calm, reassuring tone of voice.* If your voice is warm and pleasant, the patient may want to listen to your message. Alzheimer's disease patients respond to emotional tone. Your voice

should communicate support and reassurance, not anger and annoyance well into the late stages of the disease.

13. *Do not talk about the patient in his or her presence.* Even late-stage Alzheimer's disease patients have moments of lucidity. Be careful not to talk negatively about a patient to another patient or colleague. Overhearing criticism or sarcastic comments may account for at least some of a patient's negative behavior.

14. *Be realistic in your expectations.* If you are expecting normal, rapid responses, you will always be disappointed. Know their weaknesses, address their communication strengths, and be justifiably pleased with patients' honest efforts.

15. *Allow extra time for a patient to respond.* Patients with Alzheimer's disease process information slowly. If you wait for the patient to respond, you will sometimes be rewarded with an appropriate answer.

16. *Pay attention to patients' nonverbal communication.* Often, Alzheimer's disease patients cannot tell you what they mean in words, but their nonverbal communication may be very meaningful. Observe their gestures, nods, smiles, and frowns.

17. *Realize that catastrophic reactions are not necessarily manipulative.* (See Unit 10 for a definition of catastrophic reactions.) Catastrophic reactions in Alzheimer's disease patients are generally the result of frustration, cognitive overload, or the inability to communicate needs or to perform tasks. They are seldom a conscious effort of a patient to "get back at" caregivers. When a catastrophic reaction occurs, look for the cause. Examine your own communicative behavior to see whether you might have contributed to its occurrence.

18. *Listen carefully to "rambling."* Do not assume that the patient's rambling has no meaning. If the patient is talking, he or she is trying to communicate. Listen for hints of meaning in the patient's rambling. (See Unit 2 for communication changes characteristic of Alzheimer's disease.)

19. *Be willing to talk about "old times."* Relate current topics to old stored knowledge. Alzheimer's disease patients remember more about the distant past than the present. Do not be afraid to spend time there with the patient. The patient will enjoy reminiscing, and it might help him or her to perform better in the present.

20. *Continue to enjoy life.* If you feel only sad, burdened, and exasperated in dealing with Alzheimer's disease patients, you will have difficulty communicating with them. Alzheimer's disease patients are still people, and they are still capable of enjoying many happy moments in life. If you can enjoy some of the remaining moments with them, communication will be worthwhile for you both.

REFERENCES

1. Dwyer B. Focus on Geriatric Care and Rehabilitation. Frederick, MD: Aspen Publications, 1987.
2. Mateer C, Sohlberg M. A Paradigm Shift in Memory Rehabilitation. In H Whitaker (ed), Neuropsychological Studies of Non-Focal Brain Injury: Dementia and Closed Head Injury. New York: Springer, 1988;180.
3. Bourgeois MS. Evaluating memory wallets in conversations with persons with dementia. J Speech Hear Res 1992;35:1344.
4. Lyon J. Communication Partners: Their Value in Reestablishing Communication with Aphasic Adults. In T Prescott (ed), Clinical Aphasiology. Boston: College-Hill, 1989;11.
5. Clark L, Witte K. Nature and Efficacy of Communication Management in Alzheimer's Disease. In R Lubinski (ed), Dementia and Communication. Philadelphia: BC Decker, 1991;238.
6. Boczko F. The Breakfast Club: A multi-modal language stimulation program for nursing home residents with Alzheimer's disease. Am J Alzheimer's Care Rel Dis Res 1994;(July/Aug):35.
7. Santo Pietro MJ, Boczko F. Preliminary examination of the Breakfast Club: a multi-modal group communication intervention for mid-stage Alzheimer's patients. Presented at the Annual Convention of the American Speech-Language-Hearing Association, New Orleans, November, 1994.
8. Ripich D, Wykle M. Alzheimer's Disease Communication Guide: the FOCUSED Program for Caregivers. San Antonio, TX: The Psychological Corporation, 1996.
9. Lubinski R. Why so little interest in whether or not old people talk? A review of recent research on verbal communication among the elderly. Int J Aging Hum Dev 1978;9:237.
10. Boczko F, Santo Pietro MJ. Nursing Home Settings and Residents With Alzheimer's Disease: The Breakfast Club and Related Programs. In B Shaddon, M Toner (eds), By Clinicians For Clinicians. Austin, TX: Pro-Ed, 1997.

GOOD PRACTICE 12.1 IMPLEMENTING A DIRECT INTERVENTION PROGRAM: GROUP DISCUSSION

Directions: Select one program from this list of direct communication intervention programs for Alzheimer's disease patients and answer at least four of the following questions, including question 1. Share your answers with the rest of the persons in the group.

1. A memory book or wallet
2. Communication Partner program
3. A Breakfast Club
4. A conversation group

1. Program: The direct communication intervention program that I have selected is_____

_____

2. Candidates: Which patients might be good candidates for this program?_____

_____

3. Location: Where would be a good location for the program? (Think of convenience of transportation, proximity of toileting facilities, noise and traffic distractions, lighting, etc.)_____

_____

4. Scheduling: How many times per week should the program be held?_____

How long could each session be (exclusive of transport time)?_____

_____

What would be a good time of day to hold the sessions? _____

_____

How many weeks should the program run altogether? _____

_____

5. Personnel: Who could organize and coordinate the program?

_____

Who could facilitate the sessions? _____

_____

Where or from whom might you be able to learn how such a program should be conducted?_____

_____

Would you have assistants? How would you use them?_____

_____

_____

    6. Training: Would any special training be necessary for the facilitator or assistants?_____

_____

How or where could this training be obtained?_____

_____

    7. Your role: How could you personally contribute to the success of the intervention program?_____

_____

_____

What did you learn from this activity?_____

_____

_____

GOOD PRACTICE 12.2   DOS AND DON'TS FOR ONE-ON-ONE DIRECT COMMUNICATION INTERVENTION

Directions: Choose the *three* dos or don'ts from the 20 recommendations in this unit that you think would be most helpful to you personally in communicating with the Alzheimer's disease patients in your care. Today at work try each of them at least once and write below the outcome of the communication encounter in which you attempted to put the advice to work.

Dos or don'ts:

1. _____

2. _____

3. _____

Results:_____

_____

_____

GOOD PRACTICE 12.3   SPECIFIC TECHNIQUES FOR MAINTAINING EFFECTIVE COMMUNICATION WITH ALZHEIMER'S DISEASE PATIENTS

Directions: Rewrite the final statement of each of the scenarios below or state an action you would take to employ the technique named. In each case, how could the nursing assistant respond to communicate more effectively with the Alzheimer's disease patient?

Or: Use these scenarios as a role-play activity to give students an opportunity to practice and build their communication skills with Alzheimer's disease patients.

1. *Use adult language.* A patient needs his toenails clipped but has his legs folded under the chair.

Nursing Assistant: "Hey, cutie, how about giving Mama Lou your little tootsies so I can clip 'em just a smidge?"

2. *Keep your explanations short.* The patient refuses to get up to walk and moans softly.

Nursing Assistant: "Zelda, I know you're sad that your husband didn't get here, but he called this morning, or maybe last night, to let you know that he had to go to your daughter's house this morning and he'll be late. He wants you to call over to your daughter's and tell them what time you finish therapy and what time lunch is served today. Okay?"

3. *Paraphrase, do not just repeat.* The nurses' station receives a call from the patient's daughter asking whether a package of family photographs has arrived. The nurse sends the nursing assistant to check whether Mr. Miller received them. Mr. Miller does not seem to know what she's talking about.

Nursing Assistant: "Mr. Miller, your daughter wants to know whether you have your wife's photograph up on your bulletin board."

Patient: "What?"

Nursing Assistant: "Your daughter wants to know whether you have your wife's photograph up on your bulletin board."

4. *Be realistic in your expectations.* The patient unexpectedly vomits after he has had an apparently routine day.

Nursing Assistant: "George, you have to tell me where you were and exactly what you ate this afternoon. Tell me right now!"

5. *Realize that catastrophic reactions and crying out might not be manipulative.* From her room down at the end of the hall, the patient cries and cries.

Patient: "Please help me. Where's the doctor? Please call the doctor. I'm in pain. I need help. Please help me."

Nursing Assistant: (Attempting to ignore this endless annoying monologue) "Miriam, just quiet down now. You're driving everybody crazy."

6. *Be willing to talk about "old times."* As the staff member attempts to help the patient finish his lunch, the patient begins a familiar story.

Patient: "You know, life was not easy in the Depression. Tough. Very tough. My brother and I sold apples. Apples. Don't eat apples. Can't no more."

Nursing Assistant: "I know, Jack, I know. Pay attention here. Are you going to eat this applesauce or not?"

7. *Listen carefully to rambling.* As the nursing assistant prepares the patient for bed, Harry rambles on and on.

Patient: "You know Mary is such a pain in the neck. Pain in the neck. Never could do anything right. Always was, always will be. Wasn't my fault and it was over. Just like that. Mary, Mary, Mary."

Nursing Assistant: "Quiet down, Harry. You don't know what you're talking about. Everything is okay."

8. *Use touch.* The patient is clearly agitated and fidgets in his wheel chair.

Patient: "Where are you taking me, you bastard? What's going on here? I'm not supposed to be going anywhere! Leave me alone, dammit!"

Nursing Assistant: "Now you just calm down, Mr. Peters, nobody talks to me that way! There is no yelling and no cursing on this floor!"

9. *Pay attention to nonverbal communication.* The patient is bent limply forward over his food tray. So far, he has resisted

all attempts by the nursing assistant to feed him, shaking his head and occasionally raising a weak finger to his left cheek.

Nursing Assistant: (Ignoring patient's poor eating posture and hand movement.) "Come on, Joe. Eat your peas. Try some of this tasty meatloaf. I've got lots of work to do today."

10. *Use simple words and short sentences.* The patient is dawdling over his occupational therapy project in the day room.

Nursing Assistant: "Lawrence, the basic requirement here is that you complete this art project, do what you have to do in the lavatory, and get yourself down to the dining room as punctually as possible."

APPENDIX I

Quizzes

Unit 1 Quiz

Directions: Circle *all* of the possible correct answers to each question.

1. People communicate
    a. Without saying words.
    b. Less through words than through expressiveness and body language.
    c. Both as senders and receivers of messages.
    d. Best when using words alone to convey exact messages.

2. Two ways to communicate nonverbally might be to
    a. Touch your daughter's shoulder.
    b. Write your dad a letter.
    c. Hum a song while you bathe a patient.
    d. Have a heart-to-heart conversation with your best friend.

3. Nonverbal styles of communication are
    a. Pretty much the same from person to person.
    b. An excellent means of enhancing any message.
    c. Unnecessary when working with Alzheimer's disease patients.
    d. Largely determined by the culture in which a person was raised.

4. Some of the reasons we need to communicate are
    a. To get an education.
    b. To show love and acknowledge love from others.
    c. To hold down a job.
    d. To get others to do what we want.

5. In a nursing home, effective communication is important because
    a. It saves time and money.
    b. It prevents mistakes.
    c. It prevents catastrophic behaviors and reduces the potential for abusive incidents.
    d. It can help you know your coworkers better.

6. When we refer to a "common frame of reference" in communication, we mean
    a. We should place photographs of the patients' relatives in matching frames.

    b. We have had experiences that are very similar to those of our speaking partners.

    c. We share many ideas and ways of looking at things with the people with whom we were raised.

    d. The two people speaking are in similar good or bad frames of mind.

7. Which of the following statements is *not* true regarding the set of mental abilities necessary to communicate effectively:

    a. To understand one another, two people must be able to see and hear each other; this means that two deaf persons or two blind persons are incapable of effective communication.

    b. Both people in a conversation must be able to pay attention to one another; if one or both have poor listening habits, communication breaks down.

    c. Two people must be able to understand each other's ideas; you cannot explain your thoughts to persons who cannot grasp them.

    d. Memory is essential to the ability to stay on topic or add details to a story.

8. Qualities that both parties must bring with them to ensure a good communication situation are

    a. Respect and trust.

    b. Financial independence.

    c. A common language.

    d. An open attitude.

9. Openness in communication means that

    a. The door to your office is always open.

    b. Your mouth is open when you speak.

    c. You are willing to say anything that the other person wants to hear in order to make him or her feel better.

    d. You are willing to listen to what someone has to say even though you may not agree.

10. If you are an effective communicator,

    a. You will never have an argument.

    b. You have worked on developing healthy attitudes toward yourself and others.

    c. You know that no one else can "make" you say anything you don't want to say.

    d. You must have mastered all the requirements for effective communication listed in Unit 1 or it is not worth the effort.

Unit 2 Quiz

Directions: Circle *one* correct answer for each question.

1. In the early stages of Alzheimer's disease, patients
   a. Lose orientation to time, place, and person.
   b. Seldom self-correct.
   c. Cannot remember phone numbers.
   d. Lose the apparent desire to communicate.

2. In the middle stages of Alzheimer's disease, patients typically
   a. Do not seem to know when someone is speaking to them.
   b. Ask fewer questions, start fewer conversations.
   c. May lose speech altogether and become mute.
   d. Lose time orientation only.

3. Patients in the final stages of Alzheimer's disease
   a. Lose grammar and diction; speak in jargon.
   b. Lose the ability to understand what is read, although reading mechanics are preserved.
   c. Can pay attention to a speaker for a few minutes but are easily distracted.
   d. Use related words, such as "horse" for "cow."

4. *Empty speech* is very common in Alzheimer's disease patients and means that
   a. They are apt to say the same things over and over.
   b. They only talk when their stomachs are empty.
   c. They are depressed.
   d. They use vague terms such as "it," "those," and "over there" in place of specific names, such as "Doris" or "the coffee."

5. If a patient stops conversation by swearing, walking away, crying, or making rude statements, we call that behavior
   a. A window of lucidity.
   b. A violation of conversational rules.
   c. Stereotypic language.
   d. Empty speech.

6. When elderly persons lose their careers or social roles, the most common response is
   a. They feel relieved that they no longer have to put on a cheerful face all of the time.
   b. They develop xerostomia (dry mouth) because they no longer talk to people all day.
   c. They feel they are not who they used to be; to feel isolated and to feel that they have little in common with other patients.
   d. They no longer walk to activities by themselves.

7. Among elderly persons, which is the most frequent trigger for feelings of helplessness?
   a. Losing their appetite.
   b. Losing their home or familiar living environment.
   c. Losing their hair.
   d. Losing a rosary.

8. The most difficult-to-resolve situation preventing elderly persons from communicating is
   a. They cannot find their false teeth.
   b. They are too busy watching television.
   c. Their hearing aids are not functioning.
   d. Their favorite companions and family members—the persons with whom they most enjoy talking—have moved or passed away.

9. Which statement is true concerning the course of decline of Alzheimer's disease patients:
   a. Memories of long ago events disappear early in the disease.
   b. Procedural memory, or the knowledge of how to perform familiar tasks, is lost very early in the course of Alzheimer's disease.
   c. Alzheimer's disease patients quickly lose their need for human contact; the loss of desire for communication is an early warning sign of Alzheimer's disease.
   d. In spite of their annoying behavior, Alzheimer's disease patients continue to expect to be treated as adults and in fact perform better when treated with adult respect.

10. Alzheimer's disease patients who exhibit a desire for interpersonal interaction
    a. Are trying to manipulate the staff and upset them.
    b. Are liable to "tell on" the staff members who are mean to them.
    c. Will always speak and behave well with staff members who are good to them.
    d. Benefit from caregivers who use as many ways as possible to capitalize on this desire.

Unit 3 Quiz

Directions: Circle *one* correct answer for each question.

1. Elderly nursing home residents with Alzheimer's disease are likely to have
   a. Many more pleasant days than those without Alzheimer's disease because they are less prone to other illnesses.
   b. Additional communication problems from causes other than Alzheimer's disease.
   c. So many communication problems that there is no use trying to treat each one individually.
   d. A hearing loss that does not interfere with communication.

2. Speech, language, and voice
   a. Are three unique aspects of communication.
   b. Are all names for the same thing: talking.
   c. Are each different aspects of communication, and in Alzheimer's disease patients, voice is the most likely to deteriorate quickly.
   d. Are each different aspects of communication; language means how the words sound when we talk; speech means vocabulary and grammar; and voice means how well we sing.

3. Breakdowns in communication can occur because of the following sensory impairments:
   a. Dysphagia and dysarthria.
   b. Stroke and hemiplegia.
   c. Hearing loss and vision disorders.
   d. Loss of common sense.

4. Aphasia is primarily
   a. An inability to chew and swallow food safely.
   b. A disorder that requires patients to breathe with a respirator.
   c. An illness that causes patients to hallucinate.
   d. A language impairment caused by stroke or head injury that disrupts understanding and expressive communication.

5. Which of the following statements is *not* true:
   a. Alzheimer's disease patients are at higher risk than the general population for hearing loss.
   b. There is nothing that can be done for Alzheimer's disease patients who suffer from hearing loss.
   c. Even an otherwise healthy person with a hearing loss finds listening stressful and exhausting.
   d. Many persons with sensorineural hearing loss also have tinnitus; tinnitus gets worse in the presence of noise.

6. If one of your Alzheimer's disease patients has a hearing loss, you should
   a. Keep the neurologist informed about the patient's progress.
   b. Be aware that sensorineural hearing loss can be caused by drugs and carefully monitor the patient's reaction to sound and voice over time.
   c. Always stand behind the patient when you speak and use a high-pitched, loud voice.
   d. Stand with your back against the window glare.

7. Xerostomia refers to
   a. Difficulty with chewing and swallowing food safely.
   b. A hole in Xeroxed materials.
   c. A language problem often caused by stroke.
   d. A chronically dry mouth, often a reaction to drugs, that causes soreness and bleeding of gums.

8. The most common drug-related changes in a patient's ability to communicate are:
   a. Slurred speech; difficulty opening the jaw to eat or speak.
   b. A tendency to speak in short, quick rushes of speech.
   c. The use of an extremely loud voice.
   d. An improved ability to read fine print and detailed information.

9. Dysphagia, or swallowing problems, may be signaled by
   a. A wet, gurgly voice.
   b. An extended period of chewing followed by difficulty triggering the swallow.
   c. A low-grade fever.
   d. All of the above symptoms.

10. Patients with Alzheimer's disease
    a. Seldom suffer from depression because they have little or no idea of what is happening.
    b. Often have movement and balance problems that require them to pay more attention to where they are going than to what someone is saying to them.
    c. Can be "jollied" out of depression easily.
    d. Are fairly agile up until the last stages of the disease and therefore should be responsible for their own grooming.

Unit 4 Quiz

Directions: Select *all* of the possible correct answers to each question.

1. "The less competent the individual, the greater the impact of environmental factors on that individual." This implies that
   a. A patient with Alzheimer's disease might react negatively to even the smallest obstacle or distraction in the environment.
   b. The environment plays an active part in what Alzheimer's disease patients do and how well they do it.
   c. Environments can be arranged to reduce learned helplessness for individuals with cognition, memory, and language problems.
   d. New staff members, people with disabilities, family members, and volunteers will all function better in a nursing home that has a user-friendly environment.

2. Which of the following examples of physical barriers to communication?
   a. Long distances between the activities room and the patient's room.
   b. A minister or counselor who rarely visits the facility.
   c. Signs, notices, and nameplates that are written in small print, placed above eye level, or cluttered with too much information.
   d. An unwritten policy that staff may enter patients' rooms without notice or knocking.

3. Rearranging physical environments to better accommodate the communication problems of the Alzheimer's disease patients
   a. Takes administrative time and often is not worth the effort.
   b. Is sometimes costly, but many good solutions are inexpensive.
   c. Is more effective if the ideas come from direct-care staff.
   d. Is convenient because once a change has been implemented, further monitoring is rarely necessary.

4. Some good reasons to print all identifying labels in large block print are that

    a. This practice will help patients gauge distances and depth as they walk from place to place.

    b. The words can be seen more easily even when lighting is less than adequate.

    c. This practice supports patients' ability to read single words until late in the disease process.

    d. It gives the patients a good opportunity to practice their penmanship.

5. Patients with Alzheimer's disease who suffer from visual defects will also have the following communication problems:

    a. Difficulty reading the facial cues of their speaking partners.

    b. Inattention to another's speech when they are trying to walk, find their fork, or read signs.

    c. Getting as much enjoyment out of mealtimes as previously.

    d. Remembering childhood memories.

6. If you are working with an Alzheimer's disease patient who also has a hearing loss, you should not

    a. Use a low-pitched voice.

    b. Work near noisy services, such as waxing the floor.

    c. Lower the volume of televisions, radios, and paging systems.

    d. Lower yourself to the patient's eye level when you speak.

7. Poorly controlled odors and unappetizing food presentation

    a. Can be partly countered by finding ways to try to release enjoyable aromas in the patients' vicinity just before mealtimes.

    b. Make it useless for nursing assistants to try to alternate flavors, textures, and temperatures of the food when feeding the patients.

    c. Are part of being in a nursing home and cannot be changed.

    d. Can have a great impact on the Alzheimer's disease patient's interest in eating.

8. Ambient noise

    a. Is the noise made by objects or creatures that are present in an environment.

    b. Is made by ameboid friction in the atmosphere.

    c. Cannot be eliminated entirely but can certainly be minimized.

    d. Can increase easily because the noisier the environment, the louder people must speak to be heard.

9. Several ways to support your Alzheimer's disease patients' best ability to hear are

    a. To discourage them from wearing their hearing aids.

    b. To instruct staff members to approach one another when speaking instead of calling across the hall or from room to room.

    c. To use sound-absorbing materials around elevators, air conditioners, or ice makers.

    d. To schedule noisy housekeeping tasks when the patients are not in the area.

10. Some ways to overcome a patient's lack of interest in food might be to
    a. Prepare the patient for taste and texture differences with pleasant terms, such as "crunchy," "juicy," "smooth," or "delicious."
    b. Prepare the patient for taste and texture differences with warm parental phrases, such as "Let's eat our yummy carrots," or "Oooh, that's just too hot for our little tongue."
    c. Feed the patient rapidly so that he or she will not notice the bland taste or lumpy texture of the food.
    d. Spruce up the dining room with pretty plants and napkins; look through books of beautiful food pictures before lunch; encourage family members to bring in treats from home.

Unit 5 Quiz

Directions: Select *all* of the possible correct answers for each question.

1. Examples of "Cultivating a social environment that encourages independence . . . and self-expression" for an Alzheimer's disease patient are
   a. Encouraging self-expression by allowing patients to scream and cry out.
   b. Insisting that all patients feed themselves independently.
   c. Finding a communication partner who speaks the same native language as the patient.
   d. Allowing patients to wander through other patients' rooms at will because what they are really seeking is social contact.

2. Which of the following are examples of psychosocial barriers to communication?
   a. A long narrow hallway with a line of women in wheelchairs, one directly behind another.
   b. A noisy paging system.
   c. A high rate of staff turnover and absenteeism.
   d. No opportunities for patients and family members to have private discussions.

3. Which of the following are good ideas for reducing psychosocial barriers and making patients feel less isolated?
   a. Make a photograph album of direct care staff members that is clearly marked with names and shifts.
   b. Learn about a patient's personal history and refer to it frequently.
   c. Knock or call out your name or the patient's name before entering a patient's room.
   d. Complain about the patient to your colleagues so that they too are familiar with his or her shortcomings.

4. Examples of what can happen when the remaining cognitive skills of an Alzheimer's disease patient are not fully supported by staff are:

    a. Family members quickly assume the responsibility for keeping the patient active.

    b. The patient becomes increasingly isolated.

    c. The patient's communication skill declines faster due to lack of practice.

    d. The patient is at higher risk of becoming more dependent on staff members (learned helplessness).

5. The following are good ideas for developing a healthy psychosocial communication environment for your patients:

    a. Look for activities that help Alzheimer's disease patients pay attention to and care for others.

    b. Encourage them to watch more television.

    c. Encourage them to observe activities even if they do not want to join in.

    d. Place responsibility for communication on the patients by treating them coolly; let them know you are efficient, busy, and do not play favorites.

6. The Patient Social Communication Profile

    a. Assesses how social the patient is with other patients.

    b. Is against the law because it pries into confidential information about the patient.

    c. Provides information on the patient's past that can be a useful resource when talking with the patient.

    d. Can never be used with an Alzheimer's disease patient because it requires you to obtain the information directly from the patient.

7. When you assemble a photo album of the staff to share with your Alzheimer's disease patients,

    a. It is best to take group shots—that is, everyone together.

    b. Be sure to get a picture of every single person who comes to the facility in a single day.

    c. Let the patient decide whose photos he or she would like to have in the album.

    d. Take head shots of the staff members who spend the most time with the patient.

8. Some topics that staff members might wish to avoid but Alzheimer's disease patients might need to talk about are:

    a. Their true feelings about the food, certain staff members, the institutional routine, or their bothersome roommate.

    b. The confusing ending to last night's television show.

    c. Their fear of death and dying.

    d. The design of the nursing home and the layout of the grounds.

9. Absenteeism and staff turnover can be a major source of confusion and a psychosocial communication barrier for Alzheimer's disease patients because
   a Patients do not have a consistent person with whom to communicate or bond.
   b. Severe memory problems interfere with the patient's ability to remember so many people.
   c. Patients have difficulty getting used to new styles of touch, speaking, and being cared for.
   d. Staff members fail to say good-bye or to leave a memento before going; the patient is seldom afforded a ritual closing to the relationship.

10. The concept of privacy and personal space for Alzheimer's disease patients
    a. Is ridiculous in a setting such as a nursing home.
    b. Can be supported by remembering to knock, providing curtains between patients' beds, and so forth.
    c. Can be honored by remembering to say "Excuse me" when interrupting an activity or conversation, even if the patient is in the last stages of the illness.
    d. Can be enhanced by reserving private places for patients to be alone with loved ones or family members.

Unit 6 Quiz

Directions: Circle *one* correct answer for each question.

1. One often-overlooked reason for communication breakdowns between a professional caregiver and a patient with Alzheimer's disease is that
   a. The patient is hopeless and cannot understand anything.
   b. The family has probably interfered with the communication process repeatedly.
   c. The caregiver has poor communication skills.
   d. The previous shift got everyone upset.

2. The following statement is the least realistic communication strategy for professional caregivers:
   a. Work until you attain such good communication skills that you can handle all tough communication situations by yourself.
   b. Know when to ease up on yourself and take a break.
   c. Spend a little time learning about each patient's likes and dislikes.
   d. Believe that good communication encourages better cooperation from your Alzheimer's disease patients.

3. The following is a "diagnosable" communication problem:
   a. Mumbling.
   b. Talking too fast.
   c. Hearing loss.
   d. Poor listening skills.

4. If you suspect that you have a hearing loss, you should
   a. Act normal so no one will notice.
   b. See a neurologist.
   c. Wait and see if it gets worse.
   d. See a licensed audiologist.

5. Humor is healthy in the workplace; it relieves stress and builds relationships. Therefore, it is OK to

a. Tell the patients funny or embarrassing things you did as a teenager.

b. Keep coworkers laughing with ethnic jokes as long as you are sure the patients cannot hear you or can no longer understand.

c. Laugh politely when patients refer to the "inferior status" of others.

d. Share with your coworkers, in delightful detail, the embarrassing things that demented patients or their relatives have done.

6. If you are a foreign-born employee of the nursing home, you should
   a. Realize that not all communication problems that you encounter occur because of you or your difficulty with English.
   b. Make a special effort to advocate for diversity training in your facility.
   c. Make fun of the way you were raised so that everyone will see that you are a "regular" person.
   d. Assume that the other people on your shift are going to be sincerely interested in your culture.

7. Caregivers who are extremely extroverted
   a. Are always excellent listeners.
   b. Can make a patient feel overwhelmed.
   c. Contribute wonderful attributes, such as excitement and unpredictability, to an otherwise dull job.
   d. Are best suited to work with Alzheimer's disease patients under any conditions.

8. Continuing education programs
   a. Can help you integrate your daily experience with new ideas.
   b. Are the perfect answer; you cannot get enough of the new information about recent developments that might solve all of your problems.
   c. Are nonsense; you've had 20 years of experience and can usually tell the instructor a thing or two.
   d. Are a bore; how can anyone sit through that stuff?

9. An example of communicating responsibly in a sensitive situation is
   a. The time Mabel fell out of bed and you lied to the supervisor about what happened.
   b. The day Benny died and you told his roommate he had gone back to his wife.
   c. The time Adele was really agitated, and you adopted a very slow, low-key way of speaking.
   d. Using a consistent communication style no matter what happens.

10. The burdens of professional caregiving are definitely related to
    a. The number of elderly patients you have in your care at one time.
    b. How demanding your situation is at home: finances, kids, alcoholic husband, personal ambitions, whatever.
    c. Your supervisor's mood.
    d. How overwhelmed or confident you are feeling at the moment.

Unit 7 Quiz

Directions: Circle *one* correct answer for each question.

1. Cultural differences in communication
   a. Are permanent; with great effort we can reduce the barriers they create between people but never completely erase them.
   b. Rarely create communication problems between patients and employees in a nursing home.
   c. Have no place in a nursing home. The human resources or hiring department should carefully screen applicants so that everyone speaks standard English.
   d. Are not necessary and will not happen if we just try to love one another.

2. The term "culture" has a very broad meaning and can refer to
   a. Family rituals, "in" jokes, and childrearing practices.
   b. A particular corporate or workplace environment.
   c. People from a different country or religion.
   d. All of the above.

3. If an employee "goes against the company culture"
   a. That person is looking for another job.
   b. That individual does not follow the manner of dress, sense of humor, or other behaviors generally accepted and encouraged by fellow employees.
   c. That person works in a place where there is no "company culture."
   d. That employee is a hostile, suspicious person who never likes to have any fun.

4. Conflict between staff members and patients that is rooted in cultural differences
   a. Often arises because staff members have had little training in how to communicate with Alzheimer's disease patients.
   b. Is more likely to occur where staff members whose language and cultural practices are very different from those of the patients.

c. Will never happen in nursing homes that have diversity training classes.

d. Is a sure sign that the nursing home is likely to fail financially. Time to look for another job.

5. Misunderstandings among staff members who have different cultural backgrounds
   a. Always occur among individuals who do not speak the same language.
   b. Could be avoided if staffing practices required all persons from one culture to work the same shift together.
   c. Are a sufficient reason to complain to the news media about unfair hiring practices in the nursing home.
   d. Have the potential to disrupt the quiet routine required by Alzheimer's disease patients.

6. If you are an employee who speaks English as a second language, cultural differences in communication probably pose the least problem when
   a. Your supervisor gives you explicit manual instructions and illustrations for carrying out procedures.
   b. You are speaking on the phone.
   c. You are from a markedly different culture than one of your patients and that person corrects your behavior every time you are with him or her.
   d. You are interacting with a patient's family.

7. Which of the following statements is true?
   a. Cultural differences in communication do not usually affect how a person uses touch or eye contact to convey various messages.
   b. Persons from all cultures use about the same amount of space between themselves and their speaking partners.
   c. Discussion of some topics is taboo in some cultures but quite acceptable in others, e.g., income, age, personal illness or discomfort, or sex.
   d. People from the same culture rarely, if ever, have difficulty communicating with one another.

8. Alzheimer's disease patients from culturally different backgrounds
   a. Are generally too old and infirm to express their biases regarding religion, politics, or race.
   b. Mellow out and seldom find it offensive to live closely with persons who look, sound, or behave differently from themselves.
   c. Need caregivers with special tolerance and good mediating skills.
   d. Can be taught through a direct communication intervention program to inhibit any hurtful communication behaviors.

9. Some ways to foster good communication in a multicultural setting are to
    a. "Americanize" a foreigner's name to make that person feel more "American" and to counsel the person about "how we do things here."
    b. Be watchful of a foreigner's manner of communication, especially if the person is from a country that has opposed the United States.
    c. Say that you understand a person even when you do not to avoid embarrassment.
    d. Advocate for diversity training in your facility; attend these sessions and try to learn as much as possible about the cultures and communication styles of people with whom you work.

10. The most important point to remember when working in a culturally diverse setting is that
    a. You are always responsible for controlling a patient's offensive remarks.
    b. It is in your best interest to erase as much evidence of your cultural background as possible when working in a nursing home.
    c. You can always control your own responses to the culturally biased behavior of others.
    d. Alzheimer's disease patients become increasingly rude if they are allowed to get away with ethnic slurs.

Unit 8 Quiz

Directions: Circle *one* correct answer for each question.

1. Acts of psychological abuse, including verbal abuse and communication neglect, occur in nursing homes
   a. As much as physical abuse.
   b. Rarely.
   c. About 10 times more frequently than acts of physical abuse.
   d. At least four times more often than acts of physical abuse.

2. Verbal abuse
   a. Is against the law so should be used with caution.
   b. Is just a way of speaking to people in this day and age; no one means anything by it.
   c. Attempts to control a patient's behavior with violent words and actions as well as with physical force.
   d. Attempts to control a patient's behavior with violent words and gestures, but without physical force.

3. Communication neglect
   a. Is necessary when the staff becomes very busy; you do not have time to talk or to be pleasant.
   b. Dehumanizes the caregiver as well as the patient.
   c. Is necessary because it keeps you from getting too attached to certain patients and feeling badly when they die or are moved.
   d. Should never be a reason for an efficient employee's discharge.

4. Toxic talk
   a. Is irresponsible conversation about nursing home patients, events, or procedures.
   b. Is healthy; direct-care staff need to vent occasionally.
   c. Is OK as long as the wrong people do not hear what you are saying.
   d. Is a ridiculous concept; it is seldom "destructive" or "reflective of poor professionalism."

5. Which of the following statements is *not* true? Verbal abuse and communication neglect occur more readily in work settings where
   a. The acoustics are poor.
   b. Staff members are less experienced.
   c. The staff is poorly trained in prevention of abuse and neglect.
   d. Employees harbor negative attitudes toward the patients.

6. A high rate of aggression toward staff members by confused or demented patients may be a sign that
   a. The nursing home needs to hire a top-rated interior decorator.
   b. Most of the patients are from lower social and economic levels.
   c. The staff has gotten into habits of speaking and behaving insensitively to the patients.
   d. The staff is not being strict enough with the patients.

7. The possibility that you would ever commit an act of verbal abuse is reduced if
   a. You are a nice person.
   b. You had a decent upbringing; therefore, you know better.
   c. You rarely speak to the patients other than to tell them what to do.
   d. You are very aware of your emotions and know when to back off or ask for help.

8. If you witnessed what you suspected was a case of on-going communication neglect, you would be justified in
   a. Speaking confidentially to your supervisor or to the proper administrator.
   b. Keeping quiet and taking responsibility for being especially nice to the patient yourself.
   c. Asking your coworkers if they have noticed the same behavior.
   d. Going directly to state authorities.

9. A final point in this unit is that
   a. Abuses and neglect are at least as common in business and engineering as they are in the healthcare professions.
   b. Illegal practices decline where workers know that reporting abusive incidents is a fair way to deal with the problem.
   c. Many workers transfer into business and engineering careers because of dissatisfaction with abuses and neglect that they see in nursing homes.
   d. Illegal practices disappear when everyone is afraid someone will "blow the whistle."

10. It is a good idea to know and understand the law in your state regarding abuse and neglect in nursing homes because
    a. Direct care staff have a primary obligation to lecture families about the law.
    b. You will not have to hire a lawyer if you should become involved in a case of abuse or neglect.
    c. You may one day be called on to report or testify concerning a suspected act of abuse or neglect.
    d. You will know just how far you can go if you ever need to abuse or neglect a patient.

Unit 9 Quiz

Directions: Circle *all* of the possible correct answers to each question.

1. You should frequently engage your Alzheimer's disease patients in social conversation because
   a. The patient's family will think you are a nice person.
   b. Many of these patients are still capable of meaningful communication.
   c. Responding to the social needs of the patient reduces the likelihood of catastrophic reactions.
   d. It forces you to practice good English.

2. Task talk
   a. Is abrupt and rude; it should seldom be used with Alzheimer's disease patients.
   b. Is any command that tells a patient what to do.
   c. Places the patient into a passive role and fosters dependency.
   d. Is the communication style used most often by direct-care staff members with their patients.

3. Social conversation
   a. Is a healthy, natural way to nourish another person's self-esteem.
   b. Tends to be fruitless with Alzheimer's disease patients.
   c. Becomes more difficult with Alzheimer's disease patients as their cognitive abilities decline.
   d. Is a type of communication that encourages Alzheimer's disease patients to interact more genuinely.

4. Taking responsibility for social conversation with an Alzheimer's disease patient means
   a. Giving the patient enough time to respond before going on to your next utterance.
   b. Understanding that the patient may not use the correct words or have the facts straight.

    c. Opening a conversation instead of waiting for the patient to begin.

    d. Bringing up topics of specific interest to the patient.

5. You know you have had a successful conversation with an Alzheimer's disease patient when
    a. The patient eats a better lunch afterward.
    b. The patient answers you with a complete sentence.
    c. You see signs that the two of you have shared a thought or a feeling: eye contact, a nod or smile, a phrase or two in reply.
    d. A patient who has not spoken in a long while gives you an answer.

6. Choice questions
    a. Allow patients to recognize a possible correct answer.
    b. Demean patients because they make things too simple.
    c. Are dangerous to use; you should not offer too many choices to the patients, because patients might begin to "take advantage."
    d. Are not as helpful as open-ended questions, which allow patients to elaborate in any way they wish.

7. If you want to have a successful conversational exchange with an Alzheimer's disease patient, you should never
    a. Bring up your own opinions or experience.
    b. Laugh at what they say.
    c. Rely on a series of friendly affirmations ("yes," "um hmm," "you don't say") to keep the conversation going.
    d. Use only task talk.

8. The following responses are examples of repair techniques:
    a. (Patient: "I need that. Hand it to me.") "The cup is hard for you to reach; here's your cup, Sarah."
    b. (Patient: "There aren't enough pillows.") "Those aren't pillows, Jesse. That's toilet paper. Toi-let pa-per, see?"
    c. (Patient: "Abby came.") "I thought I saw Dolores in the hallway. Dolores, your daughter? Dolores has lost a little weight, hasn't she?"
    d. (Patient: "Hi, Ellen.") "It's not Ellen, honey. Remember me? I'm here on the weekends. Good ole Helen, every Saturday just for you."

9. Direct orders should be used as a conversational technique because
    a. Patients feel most secure when they are told what to do in no uncertain terms.
    b. They are just about the only way to get some patients to cooperate.
    c. They take less time.
    d. None of the above.

10. As you practice using the four conversational techniques recommended in this unit,
    a. Your own enjoyment of the job will decrease.
    b. It may be easier to deal with the residents for whom you care.
    c. You will become more skillful in using them to augment the necessary task talk.
    d. You will no longer need to use task talk.

Unit 10 Quiz

Directions: Circle *one* correct answer for each question.

1. When a patient has a catastrophic reaction
   a. It is usually because someone used poor communication techniques and upset the person.
   b. The best techniques for calming the patient might be nonverbal.
   c. You should use a loud, high-pitched voice so that the patient can hear you clearly.
   d. Refrain from using eye contact; eye contact is always very threatening to a patient.

2. Chronic or repetitive behaviors
   a. Must simply be ignored; they are a product of Alzheimer's disease and there is very little anyone can do except endure them.
   b. Are not a product of the disease but are the result of poor environmental arrangements.
   c. Can sometimes be reduced or made less annoying by changing staff responses or environmental arrangements.
   d. Have no meaning as far as the patient's communication is concerned.

3. A patient's hallucinations
   a. Can be useful if you want to demonstrate to the family or the physician how poorly the patient is doing.
   b. Should be corrected immediately by using consistent reality orientation techniques.
   c. Can be accepted by you as a moment of conversation if the patient is not upsetting others with the delusion.
   d. Can only be attributed to a toxic drug reaction.

4. When patients constantly repeat questions or phrases,
   a. Ask them to write out their questions so that you can read them later.
   b. Refer them to the bulletin board where the day's or week's activities are listed.

    c. Sit with them at least 10 or 15 minutes twice a day and talk to them.

    d. Make up a binder or a wallet with a few single words or pictures to remind them of the information they wish to remember.

5. Many times when patients resist the caregiver
   a. It is because they feel they are being treated like children.
   b. They do so with the deliberate intention of upsetting the caregiver.
   c. They have probably resisted authority all their lives; they do not know how to react any differently.
   d. It is a sure sign of an adverse reaction to drugs.

6. Resistant behavior can best be softened if the caregiver
   a. Stands above the patient's eye level and uses firm body language, such as hands on hips or arms crossed, with a serious face and a clear voice of authority.
   b. Adopts a cheerful tone of voice, a little louder than usual, and coaxes the patient with terms such as "sweetie" and "lambchop."
   c. Rephrases rather than repeats the request exactly as one way of helping the Alzheimer's disease patient understand.
   d. Avoids all body language and says the key words only one time so that the patient does not become confused by too many messages.

7. Patients who wander the facility and pilfer through other people's belongings
   a. Are often looking for where they belong or for their own possessions.
   b. Were probably kleptomaniacs before they entered the facility.
   c. Are probably exercising their deep-seated need to clean house.
   d. Seldom get past this agitated phase of their illness.

8. The paranoia over possessions that manifests itself in Alzheimer's disease patients
   a. Is completely without basis in an institutional setting; no one would dream of taking the possessions of an Alzheimer's disease patient.
   b. Suggests that they were somewhat greedy and possessive before they became ill.
   c. Is difficult for other patients; no one likes being called "liar" or "thief"; therefore, professional caregivers should use their communication skills as mediators.
   d. Is not the concern of direct care staff; security regulations should cover these situations adequately.

9. Staff members do not make as much effort to communicate with severely demented patients because
   a. Staff members know that these patients take up bed space that is desperately needed by other, more cognitively intact applicants.
   b. It is easier to speak to relatives than patients, so staff members spend all their time chatting with their patients' visitors.
   c. These patients are so sweet and easy to care for that staff members are inclined to forget about communication.
   d. Social conversation is extremely difficult with severely demented patients.

10. Some patients in the final stage of Alzheimer's disease spend much of their time crying out or moaning. Which of the following statements is not true?
    a. Patients who cry out disrupt the quiet atmosphere of the facility and affect the communication performance (speaking and hearing) of everyone around them.
    b. It is generally not worth the effort to find volunteers or professional caregivers who are especially good with these patients.
    c. Sound-absorbing materials might be helpful in damping the shrill cries of severely demented patients.
    d. Everyone who works with the patient should try some consistent types of sensory input to soothe these patients and to provide companionship in their final days.

Unit 11 Quiz

Directions: Circle *one* correct answer for each question.

1. Rather than viewing families as a resource, nursing home personnel most commonly see them
   a. Primarily as volunteers for the nursing home's fund-raising activities.
   b. As an additional source of stress.
   c. As a great way to make new social contacts.
   d. As additional patients who must be nurtured, loved, and cared for.

2. Family members most often view nursing home personnel as
   a. Potential members for their church or synagogue.
   b. Incompetent, uncaring, or uneducated.
   c. The most valued persons in the facility.
   d. People who care greatly for the well-being of their relatives.

3. Family members bring many personal biases to the nursing home. These generally include
   a. The conviction that placement in a nursing is absolutely the best solution to their caregiving problems.
   b. The idea that they no longer need to control their relative's life and environment.
   c. The guilty feeling that people go to a nursing home only when there is no other place to live.
   d. The notion that placement in the nursing home is the most inexpensive means of caring for their loved one.

4. Before being placed in a nursing home, the patient and his or her primary family caregiver have often had severe communication problems leading to
   a. Either patient-to-caregiver or caregiver-to-patient violence.
   b. A vast improvement in the social life of the caregiver, who has typically learned to find fun and relieve stress outside the home.

    c. A higher rate of caregiver enrollment in psychotherapeutic counseling with a professional.

    d. A helpful change in the time that the two people communicate best with one another, usually from late evening to midday.

5. Families of Alzheimer's disease patients must make many emotional and spiritual adjustments. Which statement is likely to be true?

    a. Typically, the person who has made the hard decision to place a relative in the nursing home is praised and supported by family members.

    b. The search for meaning in the disease is resolved by the time placement occurs; caregivers are at peace with the thought that this was "God's will" or "meant to be."

    c. Caregivers have little need to grieve further over the loss of their loved one after nursing home placement; that is why nursing home memorial services are a waste of time and money.

    d. The feelings of guilt, anger, and mourning often resurface after the primary family caregiver has released a relative to the nursing home; this is why staff members see so much need for reassurance, denial of earlier problems, and defensiveness among family members.

6. Which of the following statements is true?

    a. The personal communication problems between family caregivers and their relatives dissolve quickly once the patient comes to live in the nursing home.

    b. Communication problems between family caregivers and patients are seldom the result of clinical communication impairments, such as hearing loss, depression, and other problems associated with aging.

    c. Family caregivers' personal communication impairments can often be the source of communication problems with the staff as well as with the patient.

    d. Because family members are generally so relieved when they discover their relatives are receiving superior care, it is easy and fun to work with them.

7. Family members' perceptions of the care their relatives receive is based almost entirely on

    a. The quality of their own interactions with staff caregivers.

    b. The quality of food in the nursing home.

    c. The level of training and education of the staff.

    d. How much they are left alone with their relative when they come to visit; privacy with the patients becomes very important to them.

8. According to studies, family members tend to be most sensitive to
   a. How clean, neat, and efficient the staff appears to be.
   b. How many activities their relatives are taken to in a day.
   c. The degree to which the nursing home environment is sunny, light, and attractive.
   d. How well the staff protects the dignity and individuality of the patient.

9. Which of the following statements is *not* true?
   a. Family members *believe* that their perceptions are true and they act on those beliefs whether or not they are accurate.
   b. You, the professional caregiver, cannot be responsible for reassuring family members or listening to their troubles and complaints; your role is to get your job done for the patients in your care.
   c. Most staff members do not feel prepared to deal with the problems that families perceive and bring to the nursing home.
   d. You might reduce conflicts with the family if you provide them with clear guidelines for how they can assist in caregiving, how they should direct their complaints, and how they might take advantage of a support group.

10. Families usually do not expect you to give them advice; they just need to talk. This means that as you listen, you should
    a. Interrupt frequently to keep them on topic.
    b. Ask a lot of questions so you will get information that is useful to you.
    c. Use empathetic statements that lead people to say how they feel.
    d. Immediately report any complaint to your supervisor and other staff members so that together you can plan ways to head off troublemakers.

Unit 12 Quiz

Directions: Circle *one* correct answer for each question.

1. When patients with Alzheimer's disease are placed into a direct communication intervention program
   a. They will probably be cured of their communication disorders.
   b. Their expressive communication may get worse for a while as their comprehension improves.
   c. Their communication may improve if the program also focuses on improving the responses of caregivers and on improving the arrangement of the environment.
   d. You will not have to work so hard on your own communication skills.

2. Which of the following situations would provide the best opportunity for engaging the patient in conversation?
   a. You meet the patient moving quickly toward the bathroom.
   b. You are wheeling the patient to her next activity; she has a moderate to severe hearing loss.
   c. You are bringing the patient his or her morning snack.
   d. You peek your head into the patient's room and notice that he or she has visitors.

3. The least desirable goal for a communication intervention program would be
   a. To release the patient's early memories and encourage his or her ability to speak about them.
   b. To build the skills of individual caregivers, especially in nursing homes that have a large turnover of personnel.
   c. To develop quick and easy communication techniques for caregivers.
   d. To promote learned helplessness in the patient.

4. A memory notebook serves many purposes. However, it does *not*
   a. Help to maintain present orientation as well as early life memories.
   b. Take advantage of the patient's ability to read single words.

    c. Provide a conversation piece to which other patients and caregivers can respond.

    d. Offer the patient a chance to learn about current events.

5. The Communication Partners program works best if
   a. The volunteer has 10 months of rigorous training in communication skills first.
   b. It is operated as an "English only" program.
   c. The volunteer is able to visit the patient frequently and perhaps even see the patient through the final stages of Alzheimer's disease.
   d. The activities are planned solely around the volunteer's interests and abilities.

6. In programs such as FOCUSED, caregivers
   a. Are given instruction and role-playing practice to improve their communication skills.
   b. Earn a certificate in gerontology.
   c. Learn new skills primarily by viewing videotapes.
   d. Are assured that they have no responsibility in the decline of the communication skills of Alzheimer's disease patients.

7. Which of the following would be the least desirable procedure for an Alzheimer's disease conversation group?
   a. Prevent wandering by placing the table in the corner of the room.
   b. Reward every single effort that every patient makes to communicate.
   c. Serve some food or drink at every session.
   d. Stick to a structured question-and-answer format at all times.

8. Programs such as the Breakfast Club or conversation groups
   a. Rely on the facilitator to do most of the talking and encourage patients to interact with the group facilitator rather than with each other.
   b. Provide a central conversational theme on which the patients can focus, and objects they can manipulate, such as food, a Polaroid camera, or plants.
   c. Try to schedule at least 10 patients to a group to stimulate verbalization and increase interactions.
   d. Usually focus on orienting the patient to day, time, and place.

9. The Breakfast Club is a good way to
   a. Teach patients how to cook.
   b. Set up a strict structure for the participants so that they do not have to make any decisions.
   c. Put the patients on a healthier diet.
   d. Stimulate all five senses and allow practice of the procedural skills and social rituals that go with mealtime.

10. The direct intervention programs discussed in this unit
    a. Offer caregivers specific guidelines for trying out and then carefully examining the results of a particular way of communicating with patients.
    b. Can only be implemented by persons who are communication specialists, e.g., speech-language pathologists.
    c. Have been well researched but have not proved successful in reducing the burden of caregiving.
    d. Would never work in your nursing home.

Keys to Quizzes

UNIT 1

1. a, b, c
2. a, c
3. b, d
4. a, b, c, d
5. a, b, c, d
6. b, c
7. a
8. a, c, d
9. d
10. b, c

UNIT 2

1. c
2. b
3. a
4. d
5. b
6. c
7. b
8. d
9. d
10. d

UNIT 3

1. b
2. a
3. c
4. d
5. b
6. b
7. d
8. a
9. d
10. b

UNIT 4

1. a, b, c, d
2. a, c
3. b, c
4. b, c
5. a, b, c
6. b
7. a, d
8. a, c, d
9. b, c, d
10. a, d

UNIT 5

1. c
2. c, d
3. a, b, c
4. b, c, d
5. a, c
6. c
7. d
8. a, c
9. a, b, c, d
10. b, c, d

UNIT 6

1. c
2. a
3. c
4. d
5. a
6. b
7. b
8. a
9. c
10. d

UNIT 7

1. a
2. d
3. b
4. b
5. d
6. a
7. c
8. c
9. d
10. c

UNIT 8

1. d
2. d
3. b
4. a
5. a
6. c
7. d
8. a
9. b
10. c

UNIT 9

1. b, c
2. b, c, d
3. a, c, d
4. a, b, c, d
5. c, d
6. a
7. c, d
8. a, c
9. d
10. b, c

UNIT 10

1. b
2. c
3. c
4. d
5. a
6. c
7. a
8. c
9. d
10. b

UNIT 11

1. b
2. b
3. c
4. a
5. d
6. c
7. a
8. d
9. b
10. c

UNIT 12

1. c
2. c
3. d
4. d
5. c
6. a
7. d
8. b
9. d
10. a

APPENDIX II

Overheads

Unit 1
Communication in the Nursing Home

OVERHEAD 1.1: DEFINITIONS

Communication: Communication occurs when we send or receive messages or when we assign meaning to another person's signals. Other terms:

    Environment: Physical aspects

                      Psychosocial aspects

    Source and receiver

    Spoken words

    Expression

    Body language

Effective communication: Effective communication occurs when the message we intend is accurately understood by another person, who then replies appropriately.

Communication competence: The more ways we have of expressing ourselves, the greater the likelihood that we will be able to communicate effectively in any situation.

Verbal communication: Verbal communication consists of the actual words that we speak.

Nonverbal communication: More than 90% of our communication lies in the nonverbal realm:

Expression	Touch
Body position	Facial expression and eye contact
Body orientation	Personal appearance
Gesture	Personal environment

OVERHEAD 1.2: NONVERBAL COMMUNICATION

1. We communicate most of our information through nonverbal means.

2. Nonverbal communication can augment, repeat, substitute for, or even contradict verbal information.

3. Our style of nonverbal communication is determined by our cultures, families, and individual personalities.

4. Some people use nonverbal communication more effectively than others.

5. The ability to use and interpret nonverbal information helps us work effectively with Alzheimer's disease patients.

OVERHEAD 1.3: WHY WE COMMUNICATE

We communicate

1. To exchange information.

2. To meet our physical needs.

3. To meet our social and emotional needs.

4. To engage in self-disclosure.

5. To control; exert power; manipulate.

6. To meet the needs of others.

7. To have a therapeutic effect on others.

OVERHEAD 1.4: IMPORTANCE OF EFFECTIVE COMMUNICATION IN NURSING HOMES

Effective communication

1. Saves time.

2. Prevents mistakes; saves work later on.

3. Calms patients; calms caregivers.

4. Defuses power struggles; prevents catastrophic behaviors; reduces the potential for abuse.

5. Prevents learned helplessness in patients.

6. Reduces isolation and depersonalization of patients and caregivers.

7. Promotes personal bonding between patients and caregivers.

8. Promotes self-esteem in patients and caregivers.

9. Reduces worker stress; reduces high rate of caregiver burnout.

10. Saves facility money.

OVERHEAD 1.5: REQUIREMENTS FOR EFFECTIVE COMMUNICATION

1. A place

2. A shared language

3. A common frame of reference

4. A certain set of mental abilities: perception, attention, intellectual understanding, and memory

5. Openness

6. Expectation of response

7. Respect and trust

Unit 2
Communication Problems and Strengths of Patients with Alzheimer's Disease and Related Disorders

---

OVERHEAD 2.1: DEFINITIONS

Communication disorder: A communication disorder is a condition that interferes with a person's ability to be understood or to understand the communication of others.

Learned helplessness: "Learned helplessness arises when persons learn through repeated experiences that their actions have little effect on the outcome of the situation—especially in the 'restricted' environment of the nursing home." (S Foy, M Mitchell, 1990;1.)

Communication breakdown: Communication breakdown occurs when the listener does not understand the words or the intent, or both, of the speaker's message; *not* necessarily the result of a communication disorder.

OVERHEAD 2.2: EARLY STAGE COMMUNICATION LOSSES DUE TO ALZHEIMER'S DISEASE

Memory	Understanding	Speech and language skills	Social skills
Patients lose	Patients lose	Patients lose	Patients lose
• time orientation	• ability to understand	• ideas of what to talk about	• ability to stay on topic
• some long-term and short-term memory (not always apparent in conversation)	– rapid speech – speech in noisy or distracting environments	• ability to process language rapidly (slow processing apparent in pauses and hesitancies)	• control over anger; become argumentative
• recently acquired information	– complex or abstract conversation	• rapid naming ability—will use related words, such as "salt" for "sugar" (ability to self-correct is retained)	• "conversational bridges," making speech seem blunt and rude
• ability to retain five-item lists or telephone numbers	– sarcastic humor or innuendo • ability to process language rapidly		• ability to pay attention to speaker for more than a few minutes

Source: Adapted from E Ostuni, MJ Santo Pietro, 1991.

OVERHEAD 2.3: MIDDLE STAGE COMMUNICATION LOSSES DUE TO ALZHEIMER'S DISEASE

Memory	Understanding	Speech and language skills	Social skills
Patients lose	Patients lose	Patients lose	Patients
• time and place orientation (not person)	• ability to understand ordinary or prolonged conversation	• naming abilities, especially abstract or specific words	• lose ability to see things from another's point of view; become more egocentric
• additional long-term and short-term memory (apparent in conversation)	• ability to focus and maintain attention in presence of distraction or noise	• fluency; there are more pauses, revisions, and sentence fragments	• ask fewer questions
• abstract vocabulary and concepts	• ability to understand what is read, although reading mechanics are preserved	• ability to self-correct	• start fewer conversations
• ability to remember names of less familiar people	• some ability to read facial cues, although perception of emotional meaning is retained	• loudness of voice and vocal expression in conversation	• make less eye contact
• ability to remember three-item lists or three-step commands		• creative, "propositional" use of language	• seldom comment or self-correct
• ability to retain information shortly after presented			• lose "niceness" in conversation

Source: Adapted from E Ostuni, MJ Santo Pietro, 1991.

OVERHEAD 2.4: LATE STAGE COMMUNICATION LOSSES DUE TO ALZHEIMER'S DISEASE

Memory	Understanding	Speech and language skills	Social skills
Patients lose	Patients lose	Patients	Patients lose
• orientation to time, place, and person	• ability to understand most word meanings	• lose ability to finish sentences	• awareness of social interaction or expectations
• ability to form new memories	• overall awareness (do not seem to know when being spoken to)	• lose grammar and diction; speak in jargon	• apparent desire to communicate
• ability to recognize family members		• may lose speech altogether; may become mute	

Source: Adapted from E Ostuni, MJ Santo Pietro, 1991.

**OVERHEAD 2.5: CHARACTERISTIC CHANGES
IN COMMUNICATION OF ALZHEIMER'S
DISEASE PATIENTS**

1. Stereotypic language

2. Empty speech

3. Paraphasias

4. Violations of conversational rules

5. Windows of lucidity

**OVERHEAD 2.6: COMMUNICATION BREAKDOWNS
DUE TO THE AGING PROCESS**

1. Loss of physical and financial independence

2. Loss of livelihood and social role

3. Loss of physical attractiveness and grooming skills

4. Loss of energy

5. Loss of family and friends

6. Loss of familiar environments

7. Loss of communication partners who speak the
   same first language

**OVERHEAD 2.7: COMMUNICATION ABILITIES
PRESERVED IN THE MIDDLE STAGE OF
ALZHEIMER'S DISEASE**

1. The use of procedural memories

2. The ability to access early life memories

3. The ability to sing, recite, and read aloud with good pronunciation and grammar

4. The ability to engage in social ritual

5. The desire for interpersonal communication

6. The desire for interpersonal respect

Unit 3
Other Communication Disorders in Alzheimer's Disease Patients

---

OVERHEAD 3.1: DEFINITIONS

Speech: Speech is the way words sound when we talk.

Language: Language is composed of vocabulary, grammar, and intention to communicate—that is, putting words together into sentences to express ideas and feelings.

Voice: Voice is the sound produced by the vibrations of the vocal cords within the larynx, or "voice box," in the throat.

Hearing: Hearing is the sensory process by which sound is transmitted physically and neurologically from the environment to the brain, where it is interpreted as a message. The ear has three parts:

> Outer ear and ear canal
>
> Middle ear
>
> Inner ear

and is ennervated by the acoustic (VIII cranial) nerve.

OVERHEAD 3.2: COMMUNICATION DISORDERS RESULTING FROM SENSORY IMPAIRMENTS

Sensory impairments

1. Hearing loss
   a. conductive loss

    b. sensorineural loss

    c. recruitment

    d. tinnitus

2. Vision disorders

OVERHEAD 3.3: SPEECH AND LANGUAGE DISORDERS NOT RELATED TO ALZHEIMER'S DISEASE

Speech and language disorders

1. Aphasia

    a. fluent aphasia

    b. non-fluent aphasia

    c. global aphasia

    d. hemiplegia

    e. hemianopsia

    f. transient ischemic attack (TIA)

    e. multi-infarct dementia (MID)

2. Dysarthria

3. Voice disorders

4. Tracheostomy

OVERHEAD 3.4: MEDICAL PROBLEMS NOT RELATED TO ALZHEIMER'S DISEASE THAT CREATE COMMUNICATION BREAKDOWNS

1. Chronic illnesses

2. Drug and medication problems

3. Problems with oral hygiene and nutrition

4. Clinical depression

5. Balance and movement problems

OVERHEAD 3.5: SUDDEN CHANGES IN SPEECH, LANGUAGE, OR VOICE

A sudden change in the patient's customary way of communicating can signal a serious medical problem or emotional crisis. Be alert to:

- *Speech* that is suddenly harder to hear or understand.

- *Language* that suddenly becomes hallucinatory or deteriorates to mutism or endless crying out.

- *Voice* quality that is wet and gurgly, hoarse, or "whispery" for prolonged periods of time.

Unit 4
Effects of the Physical Environment on Communication and Recommendations for Improving Environmental Factors

---

OVERHEAD 4.1: DEFINITIONS

Communication-impaired environment: "A communication-impaired environment is one in which there are few opportunities for successful, meaningful communication." (R Lubinski, 1991;257.)

Physical environment: The physical environment includes the nursing home buildings and grounds and all the objects contained within. The physical environment also is the way space is used and decorated and the sights, sounds, smells, tastes, and textures of each unique place.

OVERHEAD 4.2: FACTORS INTERFERING WITH GOOD VISION

---

1. Poorly arranged or inadequate lighting, glaring or unfiltered light, or shiny surfaces.

2. Lack of visual accessibility.

3. Missing or inadequate signage and information display (i.e., too small, illegible print, or too much print.)

4. Too little visual stimulation.

5. Too much visual stimulation or clutter.

**OVERHEAD 4.3: FACTORS INTERFERING
WITH GOOD HEARING**

1. Too much ambient noise.

2. Lack of proper amplification where sound and voice need to be heard.

3. Not enough pleasurable or soothing auditory stimulation.

4. Lack of familiar sounds and voices.

**OVERHEAD 4.4: FACTORS INTERFERING WITH THE
ENJOYMENT OF AROMAS AND TASTE**

1. Aromas
   a. lack of pleasant aromas
   b. poor control of unpleasant odors

2. Tastes
   a. lack of positive taste experiences
   b. staff inattention to residents' tastes and food preferences
   c. unpleasant dining experiences

Unit 5
Effects of the Psychosocial Environment on Communication and Steps for Improving Environmental Factors

---

OVERHEAD 5.1: FOOD FOR THOUGHT

Although it is unrealistic to assume that lifelong social roles can be completely retained, it is possible to cultivate a social environment that encourages self-sufficiency, independence, contribution, and self-expression to the degree possible for the individual.

—R Lubinski, 1991

OVERHEAD 5.2: DEFINITIONS

Psychosocial barriers: Psychosocial barriers exist when
a. the environment and staff do not support the preserved abilities of the patient,
b. patients are not treated with regard or respect by the staff or other patients, and
c. the patient's privacy and personal space have low priority in a facility's daily operation.

OVERHEAD 5.3: PSYCHOSOCIAL BARRIERS TO COMMUNICATION—COGNITIVE FUNCTIONS

Factors affecting preservation of cognitive functions include

1. Too few activities at the Alzheimer's disease patient's level; activities too difficult for residents to access; or insufficient transportation provided to and from activities.

2. Staff unawareness of a patient's personal history; staff failure to use the family as a resource; staff lack of respect for cultural preferences and practices.

3. High rate of nursing home staff absenteeism or turnover.

OVERHEAD 5.4: PSYCHOSOCIAL BARRIERS TO COMMUNICATION—SOCIAL INTERACTION

Factors affecting social interaction include

1. Poor arrangement of rooms and furniture.

2. Unnecessarily restrictive, institutional "rules" or unspoken policies.

3. Staff members who use primarily impersonal, task-related communication with residents and who seldom take time for social conversation or quiet companionship.

4. Lack of attention by staff to residents' personal hygiene and appearance.

OVERHEAD 5.5: PSYCHOSOCIAL BARRIERS TO COMMUNICATION—PRIVACY

Factors affecting residents' rights and need for privacy and personal space include

1. Lack of private places.

2. Staff members and visitors who fail to respect residents' rights to privacy and personal space.

3. Inadequate procedures for protecting residents' personal possessions. Claims of loss or theft are not taken seriously.

Unit 6
Communication Strengths and Problems of Professionals Who Care for Patients with Alzheimer's Disease

OVERHEAD 6.1: DEFINITION

Communication style: Communication style is the set of verbal and nonverbal behaviors that a person typically uses to send or receive messages. Your personal communication style varies, depending on the people involved, the circumstances, and your communication goals for the moment.

OVERHEAD 6.2: COMMUNICATION ADVICE FOR PROFESSIONAL CAREGIVERS

1. Know your own communication strengths and weaknesses.

2. Be willing to improve your personal communication style.

3. Understand communication losses and retained abilities of Alzheimer's disease patients.

4. Believe that good communication skills increase the patient's cooperation and decrease troublesome behaviors.

5. Take responsibility for communicating with Alzheimer's disease patients.

6. Know and use the personal histories of Alzheimer's disease patients as a resource for successful communication.

7. Recognize and respond quickly to a patient's efforts to communicate.

8. Adapt your personal communication style to meet each patient's communication needs.

9. Be sensitive to changes in the patient's communication or other behaviors as a crisis-prevention skill.

10. Maintain a calm communication style, especially during crises.

11. Be willing to ask for help in tough communication situations.

12. Use stress management techniques to relieve personal tension.

OVERHEAD 6.3: POTENTIAL COMMUNICATION PROBLEMS OF PROFESSIONAL CAREGIVERS

1. Speech, language, voice, and hearing characteristics

2. Gender, status, and age biases

3. Cultural and linguistic differences

4. Personality factors

5. Education and experience

6. Situational influences

7. Response to burdens of professional caregiving

**OVERHEAD 6.4: FINAL NOTE ON THE COMMUNICATION
PROBLEMS OF PROFESSIONAL CAREGIVERS**

Communication success or failure does not rest
entirely on the skill level of the Alzheimer's disease
patient alone. Success or failure rests heavily on
your communication skills as well.

Unit 7
Multicultural Issues in Nursing Homes

OVERHEAD 7.1: DEFINITIONS

Culture: Culture consists of the customary beliefs, social forms, and material traits of a racial, religious, or social group.

Ethnic: Ethnic pertains to a large group of people classed according to a common racial, national, tribal, religious, linguistic, or cultural origin or background. "Ethnic" is a more precise term than "culture."

Company culture: A company culture determines the unspoken "rules" of a particular company that often govern the employees' behavior, jokes, and manner of speaking.

**OVERHEAD 7.2: WHAT CONSTITUTES
A COMPANY CULTURE?**

1. The vocabulary and professional language of the workers.

2. The informal or "inside" ways of expression and jokes based on common experiences of the coworkers.

3. Explicit and subtle codes of conduct that govern topics and styles of communication, dress, and staff relationships.

**OVERHEAD 7.3: CULTURAL DIVERSITY
IN NURSING HOMES**

1. Effective communication is at risk when people of diverse cultures work and live together in a closed community.

2. Often, 30–40% or more of the direct care staff members are from different countries, races, and cultural backgrounds.

3. In most American nursing homes the patients are 90% white, American- or European-born, English-speaking persons.

4. Finding compatible methods of communication is critical to a smoothly functioning environment required by patients with Alzheimer's disease.

**OVERHEAD 7.4: FOSTERING GOOD COMMUNICATION
IN A MULTICULTURAL SETTING**

1. Learn to pronounce other people's names correctly.

2. Tolerate differences in communication styles if they are effective, even though culturally different from your own.

3. Notice effective communication styles used by staff members from other cultures.

4. Trust that others intend to say the right thing.

5. Consider carefully who should counsel a coworker whose communication style is offensive to residents.

6. Support your colleagues' efforts to develop more effective ways of communicating.

7. Support your facility's diversity training programs.

8. Participate in diversity training with an open mind.

9. Do not assume that communication breakdowns occur only because of cultural or linguistic differences.

10. Do not be overly sensitive about culturally biased slurs used by patients with Alzheimer's disease.

11. Strive always to improve your personal communication style.

Unit 8
Verbal Abuse and Communication Neglect and Their Effects on Communication in Nursing Homes

OVERHEAD 8.1: DEFINITIONS

Verbal abuse: Verbal abuse is one of several types of psychological mistreatment in which one person speaks to another with the intention of causing emotional pain or controlling another's behavior through violent words.

Communication neglect: Communication neglect is a second type of psychological mistreatment in which a person deliberately avoids looking at, talking to, or touching a person as a means of withholding warmth and nurturing.

Toxic talk: Toxic talk conveys an attitude of disrespect for a person's humanity, right to privacy, and self-determination. Toxic talk insinuates that the person is not worth polite consideration.

OVERHEAD 8.2: CAUSES OF VERBAL ABUSE AND COMMUNICATION NEGLECT

1. Inadequate governmental oversight and protection of patients' and caregivers' rights.

2. Administration failure to create and enforce policies that support caregivers and residents, or that enhance the facility's working conditions.

3. Personnel inexperienced in crisis prevention and intervention.

4. Inadequate staff training in how to prevent verbal abuse and communication neglect.

5. Staff members under work-related stress, approaching "burn-out."

6. Employee history of solving problems with violence.

7. Negative staff attitudes toward the patients (e.g., the patients "are like children and need to be disciplined," "will only get worse," or "will never know the difference").

8. Staff members are repeatedly provoked by combative or verbally aggressive patients.

OVERHEAD 8.3: TEN WAYS TO PREVENT VERBAL ABUSE AND COMMUNICATION NEGLECT

1. Value and trust your own experience.

2. Do not allow "toxic talk" to poison your work setting.

3. Know your limitations; recognize your feelings and how they affect your work.

4. Develop a "buddy system" for dealing with troublesome patients.

5. Observe and learn from more experienced coworkers.

6. Know and uphold the Residents' Bill of Rights.

7. Attend continuing education programs on prevention of abuse and neglect.

8. Be familiar with the legal definitions of abuse and neglect in your state.

9. Know your obligations and rights regarding the reporting of suspected incidents of abuse and neglect.

10. Carefully evaluate the climate for reporting suspected incidents in your institution.

Unit 9
Positive Techniques for Successful Conversation with Alzheimer's Disease Patients

OVERHEAD 9.1: DEFINITIONS

Conversation: Conversation is one avenue of communication when two or more people talk to one another on a subject of mutual interest.

Social conversation: Social conversation is a style of communicating that establishes mutually trusting relationships and nourishes self-esteem. Underlying agenda: adult-to-adult communication.

Task talk: The type of communication that caregivers use to get patients to do something, e.g., "Turn over." "Here's your lunch. Sit up." "Move your arm." Underlying agenda: maintain efficient caregiving.

Institutional talk: A style of communicating defined by an attitude and tone of voice. Underlying agenda: parent-child relationship.

Conversational success: True interaction spoken between peers, lasting for as little as 5 seconds. You will be more successful in your conversations with an Alzheimer's disease patient if you

1. Watch carefully for signs that the patient wishes to communicate.
2. Accept responsibility for keeping the conversation alive.
3. Introduce topics that the patient enjoys and that are at his or her level of understanding.
4. Accept even brief exchanges as being worthwhile.
5. Stop worrying about the "correctness" or "logic" of a patient's utterances.

OVERHEAD 9.2: TECHNIQUES FOR SUCCESSFUL CONVERSATIONS WITH ALZHEIMER'S DISEASE PATIENTS

Use:

1. ***Choice questions*:** questions that contain the word "or" and give the person two choices.

2. ***Matching comments/associations*:** responses that draw from the caregiver's personal experience or opinion.

3. ***Closure*:** an unfinished sentence that the patient is encouraged to complete.

4. ***Repair*:** a word or statement that corrects the patient's error in a positive way by filling in missing information or replacing a vague term with a concrete one.

Avoid:

1. ***Direct orders*:** meeting a patient's resistance with a command. (More effective: describing or affirming the patient's feelings, actions, or words, then redirecting the behavior.)

2. ***Affirmations*:** giving brief, agreeable responses that do not give enough information to help the patient think of an answer. (More effective: Using affirmations to encourage and to soften requests or instructions.)

Unit 10
Positive Techniques for Handling Difficult Communication Situations with Alzheimer's Disease Patients

OVERHEAD 10.1: DEFINITIONS

Catastrophic reactions: Catastrophic reactions are emotional outbursts, sometimes accompanied by physical acting-out behavior, that seem inappropriate or out of proportion to the situation. The reaction may be triggered by a present event or by one from the distant past.

Irritating or repetitive behaviors: Irritating or repetitive behaviors are annoying behaviors that persist beyond the normal rate of occurrence.

OVERHEAD 10.2: DIFFICULT COMMUNICATION SITUATIONS

1. Hallucinations

2. Repetitive requests and statements

3. Resistance; refusal

4. Wandering; pilfering

5. Paranoia

6. Late stages of Alzheimer's disease

**OVERHEAD 10.3: GOALS FOR COMMUNICATING
EFFECTIVELY WHEN COPING WITH
CATASTROPHIC REACTIONS**

- Keep the situation from escalating.

- Accomplish the task at hand safely and efficiently.

- Return the patient to expected routine.

- Attempt to understand the meaning of the patient's message.

**OVERHEAD 10.4: GOALS FOR COMMUNICATING
EFFECTIVELY WHEN COPING WITH CHRONIC
OR REPETITIVE BEHAVIORS**

- Reduce staff and patient frustration.

- Attempt to understand the patient's underlying message.

- Reshape the patient's repetitive behaviors into useful communication.

- Reshape staff responses to the patient's behaviors.

OVERHEAD 10.5: COMMUNICATION BREAKDOWNS BETWEEN CAREGIVERS
AND SEVERELY DEMENTED PATIENTS

Characteristics of communication in severely demented patients

Caregivers' ineffective communication responses

Patient is mute, has palilalia, or constantly cries out.

Caregivers may isolate patient physically, talk or work over the noise, cease attempts to communicate socially with the patient, or be less sensitive to cries as genuine requests for help or signals of pain or illness.

Patient is no longer able to draw on or use information from the environment or from other persons because of severe perceptual and cognitive impairments.

Caregivers may become careless in speaking about the patient, his or her condition, or other confidential information. Caregivers may make less effort to appeal to the senses of touch, smell, or vocal intonations to carry messages that do not rely on words.

Patient has great difficulty ambulating or operating a wheelchair, or is bedridden.

Caregivers may be less inclined to make activities available to the patient or to leave normal routines and work paths to say "hello" at bedside.

OVERHEAD 10.5: continued

Characteristics of communication in severely demented patients

Patient may have rare "windows of lucidity," i.e., a moment in which he or she understands and responds fully to the situation.

Patient does not self-feed and is at risk for dysphagia due to memory or sensory deficits, or both.

Patient is very near death, although may continue to live for months in this condition.

Caregivers' ineffective communication responses

Caregivers may interpret these incidents to mean that the patient "really understands more than he or she lets on," or that the patient's inability to respond at other times is "stubbornness" or "resistance."

Caregivers may not take precautions against aspiration; may be inclined to see mealtime as a task to be accomplished as quickly (but not necessarily as safely) as possible; and may delay trays and feeding times until all other residents have been cared for.

Caregivers may avoid interactions with patient's family because "there is nothing new to report," fear of "saying the wrong thing," or inability to communicate empathy or consolation.

Unit 11
Positive Techniques for Communicating with Families of Alzheimer's Disease Patients

OVERHEAD 11.1: DEFINITIONS

Family caregiver: The family caregiver is the person in the patient's family who takes primary responsibility for the patient's affairs. One-third of primary family caregivers are elderly themselves. Nearly three-fourths are women.

Caregiver burden: Caregiver burden results from the many physical, psychological, and financial stresses that Alzheimer's disease places on family members.

OVERHEAD 11.2: PROBLEMS THAT FAMILY CAREGIVERS BRING TO THE NURSING HOME

1. Negative perception of the nursing home as a "last resort."

2. Personal communication problems of the family caregiver.

3. Long-standing communication problems with the Alzheimer's disease patient:
   a. loss of reciprocity
   b. "asynchronies"—loss of mealtime and bedtime relationships
   c. deterioration of caregiver's social life
   d. emotional scars from previous domestic violence

4. Confusion over the transition in role from primary caregiver to visitor.

5. Spiritual and emotional neediness.
   a. need to deal with feelings of guilt and sadness
   b. need to remain "connected" to the patient
   c. need to find meaning in the disease
   d. need to grieve over the slow loss of a loved one
   e. need to grieve over personal losses—time, energy, and affection

---

OVERHEAD 11.3: COMMUNICATION PROBLEMS OF STAFF MEMBERS THAT CAUSE FAMILY CAREGIVERS TO COMPLAIN

1. Failing to ask family members to help with the care of the patient.

2. Appearing too busy to provide adequate care.

3. Not being well enough acquainted with patients to transport them to appropriate activities.

4. Working for the institution and not for the family.

5. Giving the impression that too many patient care duties have been "dumped" on the family.

6. Avoiding family caregivers or disregarding their importance to the patient.

Unit 12
Direct Intervention Programs for Alzheimer's Disease Patients: Increasing Their Communication Opportunities in the Nursing Home

OVERHEAD 12.1: DEFINITIONS

Communication opportunity: A communication opportunity is any encounter between two persons that offers the possibility for "good communication."

Direct communication intervention programs: Direct communication intervention programs are specifically defined approaches to providing and encouraging communication opportunities for persons with Alzheimer's disease.

OVERHEAD 12.2: GOALS FOR SUCCESSFUL DIRECT COMMUNICATION INTERVENTION

1. Maintain as many of the Alzheimer's disease patient's residual functional communication strengths as possible.

2. Prevent overreaction to disability or "learned helplessness" from occurring.

3. Relieve the burden of caregiving; maintain the health and integrity of the caregiver.

4. Improve the quality of life and maintain the human dignity of both patient and caregiver.

5. Establish harmonious functioning within the nursing home setting.

OVERHEAD 12.3: ADVICE FOR CHOOSING A COMMUNICATION INTERVENTION THAT TARGETS PATIENT BEHAVIORS

1. Choose activities that allow the patient to practice everyday communication skills, ones that recur in the resident's daily life and that the environment will support.

2. Choose activities that match the everyday routines of the nursing home (e.g., do not center activities on a single care provider if there is a high turnover of personnel; do not work on singing if patients are required to keep quiet).

3. Choose activities that capitalize on the patient's remaining abilities.

OVERHEAD 12.4: ADVICE FOR CHOOSING A COMMUNICATION INTERVENTION THAT TARGETS CAREGIVER BEHAVIORS

1. Target communication behaviors that are likely to occur in the everyday repertoire of the caregiver and the patient.

2. Target communication behaviors that are achievable and have tangible results.

3. Match the goals of the program to the level of the patient with whom the caregiver is communicating.

**OVERHEAD 12.5: FIVE DIRECT INTERVENTION
PROGRAMS FOR COMMUNICATING MORE
EFFECTIVELY WITH ALZHEIMER'S
DISEASE PATIENTS**

1. Three programs that target the patient's
   communication skills:

   a. *Memory notebooks/wallets*: albums of perti-
      nent information about the patient that use sim-
      ple sentences and pictures and serve as
      conversation or memory devices between
      patient and caregiver.

   b. *Conversation groups*: group interaction that is
      encouraged by means of reminiscence, current
      events, games, and conversation.

   c. *The Breakfast Club*: a small group of
      Alzheimer's disease patients directed in a
      structured way to prepare, serve, and eat
      breakfast, and to clean up afterward.

2. Two programs that target caregiver communication
   skills:

   a. *Communication Partners*: volunteers, sought
      first from among the patient's friends, who are
      trained to communicate more successfully with
      the communication-impaired patient.

   b. *The FOCUSED program*: a program for family
      and professional caregivers who are taught to
      incorporate seven general principles of good
      communication when they are with their
      Alzheimer's disease patients.

OVERHEAD 12.6: DOS AND DON'TS FOR MAINTAINING SUCCESSFUL COMMUNICATION WITH ALZHEIMER'S DISEASE PATIENTS

1. Use adult language.

2. Maintain eye contact.

3. Use visual cues whenever possible.

4. Use simple words and short sentences.

5. Keep your explanations short.

6. Paraphrase, don't just repeat.

7. Avoid saying, "Don't you remember —?"

8. Use touch.

9. Do not shout.

10. Try not to interrupt.

11. Avoid competition.

12. Use a calm, reassuring tone of voice.

13. Do not talk about the patient in his or her presence.

14. Be realistic in your expectations.

15. Allow extra time for the patient to respond.

16. Pay attention to patients' nonverbal communication.

17. Remember that catastrophic reactions are not necessarily manipulative.

18. Listen carefully to "rambling."

19. Be willing to talk about "old times."

20. Continue to enjoy life.

Index